BIOHACKING SLEEP

SCIENCE-BACKED DAILY HABITS

A SIMPLE STEP-BY-STEP GUIDE TO BEAT INSOMNIA, PUT AN END TO RESTLESS NIGHTS, AND REGAIN MAXIMUM ENERGY TO AMPLIFY YOUR PERFORMANCE

NATHAN CADWELL

Biohacking Sleep
Science-Backed Daily Habits
A Simple Step-by-Step Guide to Beat Insomnia, Put an End to Restless Nights, and
Regain Maximum Energy to Amplify Your Performance

Author: Nathan Cadwell

Copyright © 2025 by Tony Neumeyer & Walking Crow Publishing

Walking Crow Publishing

718 – 333 Brooksbank Ave #307

North Vancouver, BC V7J 3V8

Canada

eBook ISBN: 978-1-988099-33-0

Paperback ISBN: 978-1-988099-32-3

Audio ISBN: 978-1-988099-30-9

Hard Cover ISBN: 978-1-988099-31-6

eBook ASIN: B0DYL247C9

Disclaimer Notice:

"Your future depends on your dreams, so go to sleep."

— MESUT BARAZANY

CONTENTS

INTRODUCTION

> *"A good laugh and a long sleep are the two best cures for anything."*
>
> — IRISH PROVERB

For years, I struggled with the relentless cycle of sleepless nights and groggy mornings. As I lay awake watching minutes and hours tick by, my energy and motivation drained away slowly. The constant fatigue took a toll on my work, relationships, and overall well-being. I tried every remedy I could find, from counting sheep and counting backward from ten thousand to over-the-counter sleep aids, but nothing seemed to work. My deep fatigue turned into a frustrating and isolating experience that left me feeling helpless and desperate for a solution.

As a researcher and writer, I refused to accept sleeplessness as my fate. I dove into neuroscience, behavioral therapy, and lifestyle optimization, determined to uncover the secrets of a good night's sleep. Through countless hours of study and experimentation, I discovered a new approach to sleep that harnessed the power of biohacking to transform my nights and revitalize my days.

Biohacking, in the context of sleep, involves leveraging scientific insights and targeted lifestyle changes to optimize your sleep health and performance. It's about understanding the intricate mechanisms of sleep and using that knowledge to create an environment and routine that promotes deep, restorative rest. By strategically adjusting your habits, surroundings, and mindset, you can hack your way to better sleep and unlock your full potential.

Whether we're talking about the little-known topic of how to lose weight while you sleep, how to sleep on an airplane, how to mitigate jetlag, or just get a great night's sleep, there are many non-pharmaceutical solutions that you'll discover in the coming pages of this book. I'll even cover problem-solving in your sleep. But most importantly, my goal is for you to sleep well each and every time you put your head on the pillow.

The problem of poor sleep is pervasive in our modern world. Studies have shown that nearly one-third of adults struggle with insomnia, and countless more suffer from suboptimal sleep quality. The consequences are far-reaching, impacting cognitive function, emotional well-being, and physical health. From decreased productivity at work to increased risk of chronic diseases, the toll of sleep deprivation is too high to ignore.

That's why I wrote this book—to share the science-backed strategies that transformed my own sleep and to empower others to take control of their nights. By the end of our journey, you'll have a deep understanding of the science behind sleep, a toolkit of proven biohacking techniques, and the know-how to create a personalized sleep optimization plan.

At the end of each chapter, I've put together a summary for you to use this book as your ongoing guide and build a personalized routine that helps you get the rest you need. Each condensed guide serves as like a short-form reference, so you can focus on what works for you.

We'll explore the intricacies of sleep science, uncovering the key factors influencing your ability to fall and stay asleep. You'll learn about the power of habit formation and how small changes in your daily routine can significantly improve your sleep quality. We'll also delve into the world of natural remedies, from herbal supplements to environmental optimizations, giving you the tools needed to create a sleep-friendly sanctuary in your own home.

But this book is more than just a collection of information—it's an invitation to embark on a transformative journey. By committing to the strategies and techniques outlined in these pages, you'll take a decisive step toward reclaiming your sleep, energy, and life, as I have. The path to better sleep is not always easy, but with dedication and perseverance, you can achieve the restful nights and vibrant days you deserve.

As you navigate the chapters ahead, remember that every small victory counts. Each night of improved sleep is a testament to your commitment to self-care and personal growth. And as you begin to experience the profound benefits of optimized sleep—from increased focus and creativity to enhanced physical vitality—you'll discover a renewed sense of possibility and potential.

So, let's dive in together and unlock the secrets of a good night's sleep. With science as our guide and biohacking as our tool, we'll create a roadmap to better rest, health, and life. Your journey to transformative sleep starts now.

1

UNDERSTANDING THE SCIENCE OF SLEEP

"The shorter your sleep, the shorter your life. The leading causes of disease and death—heart disease, obesity, dementia—have strong causal links to a lack of sleep."

— MATTHEW WALKER *NEUROSCIENTIST*

When we think about sleep, it often feels like a mysterious process that happens when we close our eyes and drift away. Yet, so much more is happening beneath the surface, a vibrant world of brain activity and bodily restoration that remains hidden from the naked eye. Sleep is not merely downtime but a crucial state that occupies a significant portion of our lives. It's a period of intense brain engagement essential for our overall health and quality of life. Before the 1950s, many believed sleep was a passive state, but research has uncovered its dynamic nature and its critical role in maintaining our cognitive, emotional, and physical health. When we understand the science of sleep, we take the first step toward reclaiming restful nights and rejuvenated days.

DECODING SLEEP STAGES

The architecture of sleep is intricate, woven with a series of cycles and stages that each play a vital role in our well-being. At the heart of these cycles, we go through two different types of sleep: Rapid Eye Movement (REM) and Non-Rapid Eye Movement (non-REM).

Rapid eye movements, vivid dreams, and heightened brain activity characterize REM sleep. During this stage, the mind engages in complex processes, such as memory consolidation and emotional regulation.

Non-REM sleep, however, unfolds in stages ranging from light dozing to deep recuperative sleep. Stage 1 involves transitioning into sleep, a light slumber that can be easily disrupted. As you progress to Stage 2, your body begins to truly relax, your temperature drops, and your heart rate slows. Finally, in Stage 3, we enter deep sleep, in which your body embarks on the vital work of physical restoration, repairing tissues, and fortifying the immune system.

Each stage contributes uniquely to our health and recovery. Deep sleep, for instance, is where the body focuses on physical repair and growth. This stage is essential for restoring energy and cellular repair, allowing us to wake refreshed and ready to tackle the day. With vivid dreams and heightened brain activity, REM sleep is crucial for cognitive functions such as learning, creativity, and memory consolidation. It's a time when your brain processes and stores information, making connections between your daytime experiences. Without adequate REM sleep, you may struggle to concentrate, remember details, or manage emotions effectively.

Disruptions in these sleep stages can have far-reaching consequences. Irregularities can lead to fragmented sleep, undermining the restorative processes your body relies on. This can raise the risk of developing chronic conditions such as hypertension, diabetes, and obesity as your body's ability to regulate stress hormones and repair tissues diminishes. Sleep deprivation can also affect cognitive functions, impacting memory, decision-making, and mood regulation. Cumulative effects of disrupted sleep stages can manifest in decreased productivity, increased irritability, and a general decline in quality of life.

You can adopt strategies that optimize your sleep cycles to maintain balance in your sleep stages. A consistent sleep schedule is paramount, even on weekends, which helps regulate your body's internal clock and promotes a natural, unbroken progression through the sleep stages. Creating a relaxing bedtime routine can signal to your body that it's time to unwind and prepare for rest. This might include dimming the lights, engaging in calming activities such as reading or gentle stretching, and avoiding screens that emit blue light, which can interfere with the production of sleep-inducing hormones.

Sleep Stages Checklist

To help you track and improve your sleep stages, consider using the following checklist:

- **Create a consistent sleep schedule:** Aim for 7–9 hours each night.
- **Establish a calming pre-sleep routine:** Include activities like reading, meditation, or a warm bath.
- **Limit exposure** to screens and bright lights before bed.

- **Maintain a sleep-friendly environment:** Ensure that your bedroom is cool, dark, and quiet.
- **Use a sleep diary** to realize, prioritize, and focus on your sleep goals.
- **Consider monitoring your sleep patterns:** Sleep tracking apps can be used to identify patterns and disruptions.

Understanding and optimizing your personal sleep process lays the foundation for deeper, more restorative sleep. This, in turn, can lead to enhanced energy, improved mood, and increased productivity. Through your sleep improvement journey, you will find that the science of sleep holds the key to unlocking a healthier, more fulfilling life.

CIRCADIAN RHYTHMS EXPLAINED

I rarely use an alarm clock, generally only when I'm traveling and have an early flight. Do you think it is possible to tell your brain and body the night before what time you want to wake up and then do it? I've done this for years, and it's something you can do as you gain an understanding of your "body clock." You can try it this weekend or on your day off if you don't need to get up at a specific time. Just look at the clock to know what time is now, and then tell yourself to wake up when you want to.

Our bodies operate on an internal clock known as the circadian rhythm, which orchestrates the ebb and flow of our daily lives. This rhythm follows a roughly 24-hour cycle, influenced by light and darkness in our environment. Various physiological processes, including sleep-wake cycles, hormone release, and body temperature, are regulated by our body's circadian rhythm. At the helm of this clock is the suprachiasmatic nucleus (SCN), a tiny cluster of cells located in the brain's hypothalamus. This master clock receives direct input from the eyes, which helps synchronize our internal timekeeper with the external world. Light exposure plays a pivotal role here; it signals the SCN to adjust the production of melatonin, a hormone that induces sleepiness, to align with the time of day. Thus, our circadian rhythm dictates when we feel alert and when we start to wind down.

The influence of circadian rhythms extends beyond mere wakefulness and sleepiness. These rhythms are critical for maintaining optimal health and performance. When they are in sync, we experience a natural peak in alertness during the day and a gradual decline as evening approaches. This alignment fosters restorative sleep, efficient metabolism, and a balanced mood. However, modern lifestyles often disrupt this delicate balance.

Exposure to artificial light, irregular sleep schedules, and travel across time zones can cause also misalignment, leading to a host of sleep disorders and health problems. Jet lag, for instance, occurs when our internal clock is out of sync with a new environment after crossing time zones. This misalignment can result in fatigue, digestive issues, and even mood disturbances. Similarly, shift-work disorder plagues those with non-traditional work hours, leading to chronic sleep deprivation and increased risk of metabolic disorders.

To counter these disruptions, aligning your daily activities with natural circadian rhythms is crucial. One effective strategy is to establish consistent morning and evening routines. In the morning, expose yourself to natural light as soon as possible. This could mean stepping outside for a brief walk or simply opening the curtains wide. Natural light helps reset your internal clock, signaling your body that it's time to wake up and be alert. As evening approaches, minimize exposure to artificial light, particularly blue light emitted by electronic devices, which can interfere with melatonin production. Consider dimming the lights and engaging in calming activities, such as reading or meditating, to prepare your body for rest.

A popular study by Czeisler et al. (1999) at Harvard Medical School demonstrated how exposure to artificial light can shift circadian rhythms, delaying the release of melatonin and disrupting sleep patterns. This research highlights why screen use before bedtime can lead to insomnia. Maintaining a consistent sleep schedule and managing light exposure helps regulate circadian rhythms for optimal rest and recovery.

Incorporating natural light into your day can also enhance circadian alignment. Try to spend time outdoors during daylight hours, even if it's just for a short break. This practice reinforces your internal clock and improves mood and well-being. If natural light exposure is limited, particularly during wintertime, consider using light therapy lamps designed to mimic natural sunlight. These can be especially beneficial for regulating your circadian rhythm and combating seasonal affective disorder.

The science of circadian rhythms offers a roadmap for optimizing your daily routines, empowering you to achieve better sleep and enhanced well-being. In understanding and respecting your circadian rhythms, you can create a lifestyle that supports your sleep and overall health.

SLEEP ARCHITECTURE AND ITS IMPACT

Sleep architecture is a term that captures the complex design of our sleep cycles. Much like the foundation of a sturdy building, healthy sleep cycles ensure that we achieve the restorative rest our bodies and minds desperately need. At the core of this architecture lies the 90-minute sleep cycle, a continuous loop through which we traverse multiple times each night. Within this cycle, we transition seamlessly between REM and non-REM sleep, each phase offering unique contributions to our health. These movements are not merely a series of repetitive patterns but are essential processes that lay the groundwork for our cognitive and physical performance.

The importance of maintaining uninterrupted sleep cycles cannot be overstated. These cycles are crucial in allowing the brain to perform essential functions that are vital for maintaining our cognitive abilities and emotional stability. While we sleep, our brain processes information, consolidates memories, and facilitates learning. This is why a good night's rest often leads to improved focus, better decision-making, and enhanced creativity. Moreover, sleep cycles play a pivotal role in supporting our immune system. As we sleep, particularly during deep sleep, our bodies produce cytokines, proteins that help fight off infections and inflammation. Disrupting these cycles, even for a short while, can leave us more susceptible to illnesses that impact our overall health.

Yet, in our fast-paced world, many factors threaten the delicate balance of our sleep architecture. Caffeine and alcohol are daily disruptors; while caffeine is notorious for keeping us alert, its long half-life can interfere with our ability to fall and stay asleep. Alcohol, on the other hand, may initially induce drowsiness but often leads to fragmented sleep later in the night. Stress and anxiety are other culprits that can wreak havoc on our sleep cycles, causing us to lie awake with racing thoughts or wake up frequently throughout the night. These disruptors fragment our sleep and prevent us from reaching the deeper, restorative stages necessary for recovery and health.

Preserving healthy sleep architecture requires conscious effort and lifestyle adjustments. Establishing a consistent bedtime routine is a foundational step. By creating a series of calming activities before bed, such as reading, meditating, or taking a warm bath, you signal to your body that it's time to wind down. This routine helps anchor your body's internal clock, promoting smoother transitions between sleep stages. Additionally, limiting screen time before bed is crucial. The blue light emitted by phones, tablets, and computers can interfere with melatonin production, the hormone that regulates sleep. Setting a tech curfew and opting for dim lighting in the evening can ease the transition into restful sleep.

Maintaining a stable sleep cycle is not solely about what you do before bed; it's also about the environment in which you sleep. Ensuring your bedroom is a haven of tranquility can significantly impact the quality of your sleep cycles. By prioritizing these practices, you can uphold the integrity of your sleep architecture, paving the way for nights of restorative rest and days of enhanced vitality.

THE ROLE OF MELATONIN

Melatonin, often referred to as the "sleep hormone," plays a pivotal role in regulating our sleep-wake cycles. A small endocrine gland in the brain, the pineal gland, produces melatonin, which signals our body that it's time to prepare for sleep. As daylight fades and darkness descends, the pineal gland ramps up melatonin production, helping to induce a sense of drowsiness. Melatonin levels rise, causing lower body temperature and reduced alertness, which sets the stage for restful sleep.

Natural ways of boosting melatonin production can be helpful in enhancing your sleep quality without relying on supplements. For example, we can limit our exposure to bright light in the evening. As the sun sets, try to create a dimly lit environment that mimics the natural progression of dusk. This can be as simple as turning off overhead lights and opting for softer, warmer light sources like lamps or candles. This gradual transition into darkness allows your body to naturally increase melatonin levels. Additionally, you could consider incorporating melatonin-rich foods into your diet, such as cherries, walnuts, and tomatoes. A handful of walnuts or a glass of tart cherry juice in the evening might be a simple yet effective addition to your bedtime routine.

Melatonin supplements can serve as a short-term solution for sleep disorders or adjusting to new time zones. These supplements can be beneficial for those who struggle with insomnia or experience circadian rhythm disruptions, like those resulting from shift work or jet lag. When used appropriately, melatonin supplements can help reset your internal clock, making falling and staying asleep easier. Many articles state that melatonin is best absorbed when putting it under the tongue to let it dissolve there.

I've used melatonin while traveling, which helped immensely with jetlag. That was, however, before I learned a new technique, which I'll get into later. However, it's crucial to approach supplementation with caution. Melatonin is a powerful hormone; improper use can lead to unintended consequences. While beneficial in the short term, relying on high doses or using melatonin supplements for prolonged periods can cause side effects such as daytime drowsiness or even disrupt your natural circadian rhythm.

It's also worth noting that the regulation of melatonin supplements can vary, leading to inconsistencies in dosage and purity.

Before incorporating melatonin into your regimen, you will want to consult with your healthcare professional to determine the appropriate dosage and timing. Misuse, such as taking too much or at the wrong time, can lead to grogginess or disrupt your natural sleep patterns, undermining the rest you seek to improve. As with any supplement, it's essential to be informed and mindful of how it interacts with your body's natural processes and use only the highest quality products.

Understanding the role of melatonin in sleep regulation offers valuable insights into how we can enhance our rest through both natural means and supplementation. Whether by making minor lifestyle adjustments or considering short-term use of supplements, melatonin provides a pathway to better sleep. By respecting the delicate balance of this hormone, we can create a more restful sleep experience, paving the way for days filled with energy and clarity.

CHRONOTYPES – NIGHT OWLS VS. EARLY BIRDS

A chronotype is your body's natural inclination toward the times you prefer to sleep and wake, dictating whether you're an early riser, a night owl, or somewhere in between. This biological rhythm is not only a personal quirk but is deeply embedded in our genetic makeup. As a result, some people find their energy peaks in the early morning, feeling most productive as the sun rises, and others thrive in the quiet of the night, their creativity and focus igniting long after dusk.

These innate tendencies can often feel fixed, like an invisible hand guiding our routines, and they can significantly impact how we navigate our days. The implications of being a night owl or an early bird extend beyond mere sleep preferences. They have tangible effects on our daily routines, productivity levels, and even social interactions.

For an early bird, the morning offers a window of heightened alertness and efficiency. This is the optimal time to tackle tasks that require focus and precision, such as strategic planning or analytical work.

Night owls, conversely, find their groove as the day winds down, often excelling in creative endeavors and problem-solving during late hours. However, this natural rhythm can clash with societal norms, leading to a phenomenon known as social jetlag. This occurs when our internal clock is out of sync with the external demands of work and social commitments, resulting in sleep deprivation and decreased performance.

Understanding and optimizing your chronotype can transform how you approach your daily life. It begins with awareness and acceptance of your natural tendencies. If you struggle to wake up early despite your best efforts, it may be time to embrace your night owl nature. Consider adjusting your schedule to align with your natural rhythm instead of fighting against your internal clock.

If possible, advocate for flexible work arrangements that allow you to capitalize on your peak productivity periods. This might include negotiating later start times or arranging your workflow to focus on high-priority tasks during your most alert hours. For students, selecting class schedules that match your chronotype can make a significant difference in academic performance.

To further explore your chronotype, consider utilizing chronotype quizzes available online. I've included some reputable ones at the end of this chapter. These tools can provide valuable insights into your sleep preferences and offer guidance on structuring your day for maximum efficiency. Taking on a personalized time management approach fosters alignment between your internal clock and external obligations, which reduces stress and improving overall well-being. As you gain clarity about your sleep tendencies, you may find that minor adjustments lead to substantial improvements in both your work performance and personal satisfaction, making each day more meaningful and fulfilling.

THE SYSTEMIC EFFECTS OF POOR SLEEP

If we lack adequate sleep, the consequences reverberate through every aspect of our being, from physical health to emotional stability. One of the most significant health risks associated with insufficient sleep is its impact on cardiovascular health. Chronic sleep deprivation can lead to hypertension, which is high blood pressure. This strain can increase the risk of developing cardiovascular diseases, including heart attacks and strokes. The relationship between sleep and cardiovascular health is intricate. As an aside, so too is flossing your teeth. Many people are unaware of how detrimental poor gum health can contribute to heart disease, but I digress. Poor sleep can lead to inflammation and stress, both of which are known contributors to heart disease.

Moreover, sleep deprivation can wreak havoc on our metabolic health. When we don't get enough rest, our body's ability to regulate glucose and insulin deteriorates, paving the way for metabolic disorders like diabetes. Studies have shown that even a single night of inadequate sleep can induce a prediabetic state in otherwise healthy individuals. This metabolic disruption is partially due to the hormonal imbalances caused by sleep deprivation, which can lead to increased appetite and weight gain. Over time, the accumulation of these effects can significantly elevate the risk of developing type 2 diabetes.

The physical, cognitive, and emotional toll of sleep deprivation can include heightened anxiety and even depression. Our brains rely on sleep to process information, consolidate memories, and regulate emotions. Without enough sleep, we experience impaired decision-making, reduced attention span, and foggy thinking. This can lead to mistakes at work, poor judgment, and increased susceptibility to accidents. It becomes a vicious cycle: anxiety can disrupt sleep, and lack of sleep can exacerbate anxiety, creating a loop that is difficult to break. This cycle affects our mood, which can strain relationships and diminish our quality of life.

A well-known study by Van Dongen et al. (2003) at the University of Pennsylvania found that individuals who slept only 6 hours per night for two weeks performed as poorly on cognitive tasks as those who had been awake for 24 hours straight. Despite feeling "adapted" to less sleep, their cognitive decline continued, demonstrating that the brain does not fully adjust to chronic sleep loss.

Another landmark study by Matthew Walker (2017) revealed that sleep deprivation weakens the immune system, increases the risk of heart disease, and disrupts emotional regulation. Sleep loss has also been linked to an increased risk of Alzheimer's disease, as shown by research from the National Institutes of Health (2013), which found that deep sleep helps clear beta-amyloid, a toxic protein associated with cognitive decline.

Beyond health risks, sleep deprivation impairs decision-making, slows reaction time, and decreases productivity, making it a significant factor in workplace and driving accidents. These studies highlight the critical need for sufficient sleep to maintain cognitive function, emotional stability, and long-term health.

As mentioned, sleep also plays a crucial role in maintaining a robust immune system. During sleep, the body produces and releases cytokines, proteins that target infection and inflammation. Without sufficient sleep, the production of these protective proteins decreases, leaving us more vulnerable to illnesses. An inadequate amount of sleep can lead to a weakened immune response, making us more susceptible to catching colds and infections. This reduced immunity can have long-term consequences, potentially increasing the risk of chronic health conditions.

Although I rarely get sick, when I do, it usually gets back to being run down and several days of no sleep for whatever reason. Even with all the techniques in this book, I occasionally overdo it and burn the candle at both ends, as the saying goes. When I do, that's when I'm most likely to get a cold or the flu.

By making conscious choices to improve our sleep, we can protect our physical health, enhance our cognitive function, and bolster our emotional well-being. In doing so, we pave the way for a healthier, more balanced life where the benefits of restful nights are felt through every waking moment.

Summary:

- **Follow a Consistent Sleep Schedule** – Go to bed and wake up at the same time daily to regulate your body's internal clock and improve sleep quality.
- **Limit Evening Light Exposure** – Avoid screens at least an hour before bed and dim indoor lighting to support natural melatonin production.
- **Align with Your Circadian Rhythm** – Get morning sunlight exposure and maintain a steady routine to enhance sleep-wake cycles.
- **Be Mindful of Stimulants and Alcohol** – Avoid caffeine in the afternoon and limit alcohol, as both can disrupt sleep quality.

- **Use a Relaxing Pre-Sleep Routine** – Engage in calming activities like reading or meditation to signal your body that it's time to sleep.
- **Prioritize Sleep for Overall Health**—Chronic sleep loss weakens immunity, impairs focus, and increases the risk of heart disease and diabetes. Protect your sleep as a core health habit.

2

BUILDING A SLEEP-INDUCING ENVIRONMENT

> *"A quiet, comfortable bedroom is the foundation of restorative sleep. Control your environment, and you control your sleep."*
>
> — ARIANNA HUFFINGTON (*FOUNDER OF THE SLEEP REVOLUTION*)

I magine stepping into a room that instantly embraces you with a sense of calm. The colors soothe your eyes, the air carries a gentle, relaxing scent, and the soft hum of nature sounds lull you into tranquility. This is the essence of a sleep sanctuary—a space designed to nurture rest and rejuvenation. It's about transforming your bedroom into a haven that supports the natural rhythms of sleep and promotes a peaceful state of mind. Creating such an environment can significantly influence your ability to fall asleep and stay asleep, ultimately leading to more productive days.

DESIGNING YOUR SLEEP SANCTUARY

The colors that envelop your space are pivotal in shaping your mood and relaxation. According to research, certain hues can enhance your sleep quality by inducing a sense of calm. Soft blues and greens are particularly effective in this regard. These colors are reminiscent of serene skies and lush landscapes, evoking a sense of peace and comfort that can ease stress and create a restful atmosphere. Blue, known for its soothing properties, helps reduce heart rate and blood pressure, setting the stage for a good night's sleep. Green, associated with nature, promotes relaxation and a sense of tranquility. In contrast, vibrant colors like reds and oranges are best avoided in the bedroom, as they tend to stimulate the brain, potentially making it harder to unwind. By choosing calming tones for your walls, bedding, and decor, you can foster an environment that encourages relaxation and restfulness.

A clutter-free space further enhances the sense of serenity needed for sleep. When your room is tidy and organized, it becomes a sanctuary free from distractions and stressors. Minimalist decor, characterized by clean lines and simple aesthetics, can help achieve this calming effect. Reducing visual noise allows your mind to focus on the present moment, making it easier to relax and drift into sleep. Consider incorporating organized storage solutions, such as baskets or shelves, to keep items out of sight and maintain a neat environment. This approach not only adds to the aesthetic appeal of your space but also contributes to a more peaceful mindset.

SCENTS THAT HELP YOU SLEEP

A growing body of research supports the idea that certain scents can promote relaxation and improve sleep quality. Aromatherapy, the practice of using essential oils for therapeutic benefits, has been shown to reduce stress, calm the nervous system, and facilitate deeper, more restful sleep.

One of the most widely studied scents for sleep is lavender. A study by Goel et al. (2005) at Wesleyan University found that participants who inhaled lavender oil before bedtime experienced increased slow-wave sleep, the deepest and most restorative phase of the sleep cycle. Additionally, they reported feeling more refreshed on waking. Similarly, a study published in the *Journal of Alternative and Complementary Medicine* (2015) demonstrated that lavender aromatherapy significantly reduced insomnia and improved sleep quality in individuals with anxiety disorders.

Another scent with sleep-promoting properties is chamomile. Research from the University of Pennsylvania (2011) found that chamomile extract reduced symptoms of generalized anxiety disorder, indirectly improving sleep patterns by reducing nighttime restlessness. Bergamot, a citrus-scented essential oil, has also been shown to lower heart rate and blood pressure, creating a calm state ideal for falling asleep, according to a study in the *Journal of Clinical Psychopharmacology* (2013).

Incorporating these scents into a bedtime routine—whether through diffusers, pillow sprays, or warm baths—can enhance relaxation and improve sleep quality. While aromatherapy isn't a cure for chronic sleep disorders, scientific evidence suggests it can be a valuable, natural tool for creating a more sleep-inducing environment.

SOUNDSCAPES THAT HELP YOU SLEEP

Soundscapes, or ambient audio environments, have been scientifically shown to promote relaxation and improve sleep quality. By masking disruptive noises and creating a calming atmosphere, specific sounds can help the brain transition into restful states.

One of the most effective soundscapes for sleep is white noise. A study by Stanchina et al. (2005) published in *Sleep Medicine* found that white noise significantly reduced participants' time to fall asleep, especially in noisy environments. By creating a consistent auditory backdrop, white noise helps mask sudden sounds, such as traffic or household disturbances, which might otherwise interrupt sleep.

Nature sounds, such as rain, ocean waves, or rustling leaves, have also been shown to promote deeper rest. A study by Annerstedt et al. (2013) published in *The International Journal of Environmental Research and Public Health* found that listening to natural soundscapes reduced stress and lowered cortisol levels, making it easier for individuals to fall asleep. These sounds' rhythmic, non-intrusive quality helps signal to the brain that it's time to relax.

Another popular option is pink noise, which is similar to white noise but has a lower, more balanced frequency. A study in *Frontiers in Human Neuroscience* (2017) found that pink noise improved sleep quality and enhanced memory retention by synchronizing with the brain's slow-wave activity during deep sleep.

Incorporating soundscapes into a bedtime routine—whether through apps, white noise machines, or recordings—can create a more sleep-conducive environment. While not a cure for chronic sleep issues, the science supports soundscapes as an effective, natural aid for better rest.

Design Your Sleep Sanctuary Checklist

Use this checklist to create your personal sleep sanctuary:

- Choose calming colors like blues and greens for walls and decor.
- Maintain a clutter-free space with minimalist decor and organized storage.
- Introduce relaxing scents, such as lavender, in the form of essential oils.
- Incorporate soundscapes like white noise or nature sounds to enhance tranquility.

Thoughtfully integrating these elements transforms your bedroom into a serene escape that fosters deep, restorative sleep.

THE IDEAL SLEEP TEMPERATURE

Sleep science is closely tied to the body's natural ability to regulate temperature. As night falls and you prepare for rest, your core body temperature begins to drop, signaling to your body that it's time to wind down. This natural cooling process is essential for transitioning through the various stages of sleep, particularly the deep sleep phases, where the most restorative activities occur. When your body temperature decreases, it facilitates the release of sleep-inducing hormones, helping you drift into a peaceful slumber. Conversely, suppose your sleep environment is too warm. In that case, it can interfere with this delicate process, leading to restlessness and frequent awakenings. Creating a sleep environment that aligns with your body's needs is crucial to support natural thermoregulation.

Finding the optimal temperature for sleep can make a significant difference in the quality of your rest. Research suggests that a bedroom temperature between 60–67 degrees Fahrenheit (15.5–19.5 degrees Celsius) is ideal for most people. This range supports the body's cooling process while providing a comfortable environment that isn't too chilly.

Be sure to consider seasonal variations and personal comfort when setting your nighttime thermostat. During warmer months, you might need to adjust your cooling systems; while in colder seasons, ensuring your room doesn't dip too low is key to maintaining a cozy yet comfortable sleep setting. By fine-tuning your bedroom climate, you can enhance the quality of your sleep, making it easier to fall asleep and stay asleep through the night.

Achieving and maintaining the right temperature doesn't have to be complicated. Simple adjustments can make a world of difference. Utilizing fans or air conditioning units can help circulate air and keep your room cool, even on the hottest nights. Additionally, consider adjusting your window treatments to enhance insulation. Heavy curtains or thermal blinds can block out heat during the day and retain warmth during cooler nights, contributing to a stable sleep environment. If you live in an area with fluctuating temperatures, investing in a programmable thermostat allows you to set specific temperatures for different times, ensuring that your room is always in the perfect setting for sleep.

By prioritizing a comfortable sleep temperature, you pave the way for deeper, more restorative slumber, ultimately boosting your energy levels and productivity during waking hours.

THE BEST BEDDING MATERIALS FOR BETTER SLEEP

The materials you sleep on play a crucial role in sleep quality, affecting everything from body temperature regulation to overall comfort. Scientific studies have shown that choosing the right bedding can significantly improve rest by promoting better thermoregulation and reducing discomfort.

What you sleep on can make a huge difference in regulating your temperature. Research from Haghayegh et al. (2019) in *Sleep Medicine Reviews* highlights the importance of maintaining an optimal sleep temperature, suggesting that materials like cotton and linen, which are breathable and moisture-wicking, can help prevent overheating. Bamboo fabric, known for its softness and natural cooling properties, has also gained popularity for its ability to regulate temperature and keep sleepers dry throughout the night.

In contrast, materials like polyester and other synthetic fibers tend to trap heat and moisture, increasing the risk of night sweats and disrupted sleep. A study from the National Sleep Foundation indicates that people who sleep in cooler environments with breathable bedding experience deeper, more restorative sleep cycles.

Wool bedding has been shown to improve sleep in colder climates by maintaining warmth without overheating. A study from the University of Sydney (2011) found that wool's natural insulation properties helped regulate body temperature, leading to longer periods of deep sleep.

Equally important is choosing hypoallergenic bedding, especially for those sensitive to allergens. Materials like organic cotton can reduce allergens and minimize sleep disruptions caused by allergies or skin irritation. Silk, known for its smooth texture and moisture-wicking properties, is naturally resistant to mold and mildew, making it an excellent option for a clean sleeping environment. Silk and organic cotton feel luxurious, and they help reduce exposure to dust mites and other common allergens that can disrupt sleep. Given all the materials available, hypoallergenic bedding creates a healthier sleep environment that minimizes irritants and promotes uninterrupted rest.

Understanding the dynamics that temperature and bedding materials have on sleep empowers you to make informed choices about your sleeping environment. Invest in high-quality, breathable, and temperature-regulating bedding as simple yet effective way to improve sleep quality.

Many people underestimate the impact of a good mattress. Still, it's essential to maintain the natural alignment of your spine throughout the night. Memory foam mattresses are popular for their ability to contour to the body's shape, providing personalized support that can alleviate pressure points. This adaptive quality evenly distributes body weight, which is particularly beneficial for those with joint or back pain. In contrast, innerspring mattresses, which use coils for support, can offer a firmer feel with a more traditional sleep surface. They provide excellent support and breathability, which can help regulate body temperature during sleep. Choosing the right mattress is a personal decision, and it's worth taking the time to find one that meets your individual needs for comfort and support.

Pillows, often overshadowed by mattresses, are equally vital in ensuring spinal health and overall sleep quality. The right pillow can prevent neck and back pain by maintaining proper spinal alignment. Side sleepers will want to consider contour pillows, which are designed with an ergonomic shape that supports the natural curve of the neck. This reduces strain and promotes a neutral spine position. Back sleepers might benefit from medium-thickness pillows that cradle the head without pushing it too far forward. On the other hand, stomach sleepers should opt for thinner pillows to keep the neck from arching unnaturally. Selecting a pillow that complements your sleep position can greatly enhance comfort and prevent morning stiffness or discomfort.

Maintaining bedding hygiene includes regularly washing your bed linens, sheets, and pillowcases at least once a week in hot water to eliminate a buildup of allergens and bacteria. Mattress protectors can add an extra layer of defense, shielding your mattress from spills, allergens, and dust mites. Don't forget to wash your pillows every few months, as they can also harbor allergens and lose their supportive properties over time. Making these practices a regular part of your routine ensures a clean, comfortable, and inviting sleep environment.

The choices you make about your bedding might seem small, but they can notably impact your sleep quality and overall health. Investing in a supportive mattress and pillow, opting for hypoallergenic materials, and maintaining cleanliness are all steps toward creating a sleep environment that supports restful, rejuvenating sleep. As you align your sleep space to your body's natural needs, pay attention to how these changes affect your comfort and well-being, and then adjust as needed to find the perfect combination that works for you.

THE POWER OF DARKNESS

As nightfall approaches, the absence of light plays a pivotal role in preparing your body for restful sleep. As I've discussed, darkness is another natural cue that signals the body to begin winding down, primarily through melatonin production. This process helps regulate your sleep-wake cycle, making falling and staying asleep easier. However, artificial light has become an omnipresent disruptor in our modern world, often delaying melatonin production and, consequently, sleep onset. The glow of streetlights, the flicker of a television, or even the subtle glow from a digital clock can interfere with your body's natural rhythm, prolonging the time it takes to drift into slumber.

Creating an environment that limits light exposure as bedtime approaches is crucial. One effective strategy is to invest in blackout curtains, which can significantly reduce how much light enters your room, creating a darkened oasis conducive to sleep. These heavy drapes or blinds can block out unwanted external light sources, such as streetlights or early morning sunshine, allowing your body to maintain its natural rhythm without interruption. In addition to curtains, eye masks can serve as a portable solution, offering a personal cocoon of darkness regardless of your surroundings. By eliminating light exposure, you give your body the signal it needs to produce melatonin, facilitating a smoother transition into sleep.

Electronic devices are another source of light pollution that can disrupt your sleep. The screens of phones, tablets, and computers emit blue light, suppressing melatonin production more than any other type of light. This can make falling asleep more challenging and result in poorer sleep quality.

To mitigate sleep-quality risks, consider using blue light filtering apps or screen protectors that reduce the amount of blue light emitted by your devices. You can also adjust other nighttime light sources, such as seen with digital clocks, to their lowest level, if you have them on at all. These choices help you to minimize lighting impacts on your sleep cycle, especially when device use is unavoidable though the night. Additionally, adopting a habit of powering down screens at least an hour before bedtime can give your body the chance to wind down and prepare for rest naturally.

Creating a naturally dark environment can also enhance your sleep quality. Installing blackout curtains is one of the most effective ways to block light from entering your room. Soundproof blackout curtains are available, which will also help you to reduce noise in your sleeping area.

Simple actions like dimming the lights in your home as the evening progresses can help mimic the natural transition from day to night. Consider using dimmable lamps or even candles to light your space in the hours leading up to sleep, fostering a calm and tranquil atmosphere. By gradually reducing light exposure, you align your environment with your body's internal clock, promoting a sense of relaxation and readiness for sleep.

These steps, though seemingly small, can fully impact your ability to achieve deep, restorative sleep. By managing your light exposure and embracing the natural power of darkness, you create an environment that supports the body's innate sleep processes. As darkness envelops your room, you open the door to a night of peaceful, uninterrupted slumber, ultimately paving the way for more energized and productive days.

NOISE CONTROL TECHNIQUES

Noise can be a formidable enemy in the battle for quality sleep. Even when you think you're used to the sounds of the city or the late-night comings and goings of neighbors, these noises can subtly disrupt your sleep cycles. Imagine drifting off, only to be jolted awake by the sudden blare of a car horn or the clatter of a garbage truck. Each interruption chips away at the restorative power of sleep, leaving you feeling groggy and irritable the next day. It's not just the problematic loud noises; even low-level noise, like the hum of a refrigerator or distant traffic, can keep your brain from reaching the deeper stages of sleep it desperately needs.

To combat these disruptions, consider soundproofing your bedroom to create a sanctuary of silence. As mentioned above, installing soundproof curtains is one of the most effective ways to do this. These heavy drapes block out light and absorb sound, thus reducing the intrusion of external noise.

If you find yourself dealing with particularly noisy surroundings, you might explore further soundproofing methods, like adding acoustic panels to your walls or using door sweeps to seal gaps. Another strategy is to use rugs and carpets, which can significantly dampen sound by absorbing vibrations from footsteps and other indoor disturbances. Minimizing noise interruptions gives your mind the quiet it needs to rest fully and deeply.

These techniques may seem like minor adjustments, but their impact on your sleep quality can be quite meaningful. By controlling the auditory environment of your bedroom, you pave the way for a deeper, more restorative sleep experience. This, in turn, can lead to improved mood and increased productivity, as your mind and body are better equipped to face the challenges of the day ahead.

TECHNOLOGY AND SLEEP

Technology has become an inseparable part of our lives, providing convenience and connectivity like never before. Yet, it often plays a disruptive role when it comes to sleep. The constant barrage of notifications and alerts from our devices keeps us tethered to a state of alertness, making it difficult to wind down. Each ping or vibration can pull you back from the brink of slumber, reawakening your mind and breaking your rhythm of relaxation. The light from screens before bed, for example, tricks the brain into perceiving this artificial light as daylight, delays sleep onset, leaves you tossing and turning long after you've turned off your devices.

To cultivate healthier sleep habits, consider implementing guidelines for responsible technology use. One effective strategy is to set device curfews, which involves switching off screens at least an hour before bedtime. This allows your mind to disconnect from the digital world and transition into rest mode. Creating a tech-free zone in your bedroom can further enhance this effect. Removing electronic devices from your sleep environment establishes a physical boundary that reinforces the bedroom as a space dedicated solely to rest and relaxation. This helps reduce exposure to disruptive light and minimizes distractions that can keep your mind active when it should be winding down.

While it may seem paradoxical, technology can support better sleep when used mindfully. A variety of apps are designed to promote restful slumber rather than hinder it. Sleep cycle tracking apps, for instance, provide insights into your sleep patterns, helping you identify areas for improvement. These apps often use the accelerometer in your phone to monitor movements during sleep, offering a detailed analysis of your sleep stages and quality.

Additionally, relaxation and meditation apps offer guided sessions to calm your mind and prepare your body for sleep. We will cover mindfulness and meditation in depth through the next chapter, but here we want to think about technology-based apps and how they can help you achieve a more restful sleep. These apps include everything from breathing exercises to soothing soundscapes, or calming voice to ambient sounds, all of which can provide a structured way to ease into the night. These audio aids can be particularly helpful if you find your mind racing at bedtime, as they offer a focal point to redirect your thoughts away from stress and toward calm.

Moreover, smart home technology introduces new ways to enhance your sleep environment. Smart thermostats, for example, allow you to precisely control the temperature of your bedroom, aligning it with the optimal range for sleep. Smart lighting systems can also be used and tailored to mimic natural light patterns, gradually dimming as bedtime approaches and simulating sunrise in the morning. This helps maintain your circadian rhythm, promoting a more natural sleep-wake cycle.

The intersection of technology and sleep is a balancing act. While gadgets can quickly become barriers to restful sleep, they can also be powerful allies when used with intention. When it comes to these newer innovations, you can harness their benefits while mitigating their drawbacks by consciously choosing how and when to interact with technology. This thoughtful approach improves sleep quality and enhances your overall well-being, creating a harmonious relationship between the digital and the natural. As you explore these strategies, remember that small changes can significantly improve how you sleep and, consequently, how you live.

Summary:

- **Design a Calming Sleep Space** – To reduce stress and promote relaxation, use soothing colors like soft blues and greens, keep your room free from clutter, and opt for minimalist decor.
- **Control Room Temperature** – Maintain your bedroom temperature between 60–67°F (15.5–19.5°C) to support your body's natural cooling process for deeper, restorative sleep.
- **Invest in Sleep-Friendly Bedding** – Choose breathable materials like cotton, linen, or bamboo to regulate temperature. Use supportive mattresses and pillows that suit your sleep position.

- **Use Aromatherapy for Relaxation** – Scents like lavender, chamomile, and bergamot can promote calm and improve sleep quality. Use essential oil diffusers, pillow sprays, or scented baths.
- **Incorporate Soothing Sounds** – Use white, pink, or nature sounds to mask disruptive noises and create a calming sleep environment. Apps or white noise machines can help.
- **Minimize Light Exposure** – Install blackout soundproof curtains, dim lights in the evening, and avoid screens at least an hour before bed to support melatonin production.
- **Leverage Technology Mindfully** – Use sleep-tracking apps, smart thermostats, and meditation apps to improve your sleep routine, but establish a tech curfew to reduce blue light exposure.

3

MASTERING MINDFULNESS AND RELAXATION TECHNIQUES

"Mindfulness is the gateway to restful sleep; when the mind quiets, the body follows."

— JON KABAT-ZINN *(FOUNDER OF MINDFULNESS-BASED STRESS REDUCTION)*

In this chapter, I'll discuss several options for helping you sleep. As you read through these different methods, you'll likely find some that feel like a perfect fit, while others may not be for you. Keep in mind the personal benefits of being flexible; this book is about personalizing a routine that works for you. Try a few of these methods to determine what's best for you.

MANAGING SLEEP ANXIETY – IS THIS YOU?

As the day winds down and you retreat to your bedroom sanctuary, a familiar unease may creep in—the anxiety surrounding sleep. This anxiety is not uncommon and often stems from various sources. For many, it begins with the fear of insomnia itself. In this vicious cycle, the worry of not sleeping becomes the very thing that keeps you awake. The anticipation of another night of tossing and turning can weigh heavily on the mind, creating a sense of lingering dread at the edges of your consciousness. Additionally, the pressure of impending tasks and responsibilities waiting for you on the other side of sleep can amplify this anxiety. The mind races with thoughts of meetings, deadlines, and obligations, making it difficult to find peace as you lay in bed.

To address sleep anxiety effectively, it's essential to adopt practical strategies to help break these worry patterns. Cognitive reframing techniques can be instrumental in this regard. This involves consciously changing the narrative in your mind, shifting from negative thoughts about sleep to more positive or neutral ones. Instead of fixating on the fear of not sleeping, remind yourself that rest in any form is beneficial and that your bed is a place of comfort and relaxation. This simple change in perspective can reduce the pressure you place on yourself, easing the transition into sleep.

Additionally, consider incorporating journaling into your nightly routine. Before settling in for the night, take a few moments to write down any worries or tasks occupying your mind. Then you can relax in knowing that your thoughts will be there in the morning. By transferring these concerns onto paper, you create mental space, allowing your mind to release its grip on them, at least temporarily.

Anxiety's impact on sleep quality is significant, often leading to disrupted sleep patterns or even insomnia. When anxiety takes hold, it activates the body's stress response, releasing hormones like cortisol that keep you alert and awake. This heightened state of arousal can make it challenging to fall asleep, and even if you do, the quality of your rest may be compromised. The mind may continue to process stressors throughout the night, leading to fragmented sleep and frequent awakenings. Over time, this pattern can erode your sleep quality, affecting your mood, energy levels, and overall well-being. Recognizing the role anxiety plays in your sleep can be the first step toward addressing it and restoring restful nights.

In managing sleep anxiety, self-compassion and patience are invaluable allies. It's crucial to remember that overcoming anxiety is not an overnight process, and setbacks are a natural part of progress. Be gentle with yourself during this journey, acknowledging that anxiety is a common human experience and not a personal failure. Practice kindness toward yourself, allowing room for mistakes and growth. Celebrate small victories, like a night of improved sleep or a successful use of a new technique. This attitude of self-compassion can reduce the pressure you place on yourself, making it easier to navigate the ups and downs of managing sleep anxiety. You can create a supportive internal environment that encourages healing and resilience by fostering patience and understanding.

Incorporating these practices into your routine can gradually transform your relationship with sleep, turning anxiety into calm and worry into restfulness.

MINDFULNESS MAY BE YOUR KEY

Imagine a scene where the day's chaos gradually fades away, replaced by a serene calmness that envelops you as you prepare for sleep. This tranquility is not an elusive dream but a reality within reach, thanks to mindfulness. Mindfulness, a practice rooted in ancient traditions, empowers you to focus on the present moment, allowing your mind to release the anxieties and stresses accumulated throughout the day. Unlike other relaxation methods, mindfulness is not about clearing the mind or achieving a state of trance; it's about cultivating awareness and acceptance of the current moment without judgment. By embracing mindfulness, you learn to observe your thoughts and feelings as they are, without attachment or resistance. This can significantly alleviate pre-sleep anxiety and pave the way for restful slumber.

Mindfulness offers a myriad of benefits for sleep. When you practice mindfulness, you train your brain to shift its focus away from the relentless stream of worries and thoughts that often invade your mind at bedtime. This shift creates mental space, allowing you to approach sleep with a sense of calm and readiness. By letting go of the day's stresses and future anxieties, you enable your body to relax and naturally transition into sleep. Studies suggest that mindfulness practices can improve sleep quality by reducing insomnia symptoms and enhancing overall sleep efficiency.

A landmark study by Black et al. (2015) published in *JAMA Internal Medicine* found that participants who completed a six-week mindfulness meditation program experienced significantly less insomnia, fatigue, and depression compared to those who followed a standard sleep education program. The mindfulness group reported improved sleep quality due to reduced pre-sleep arousal and racing thoughts, common contributors to insomnia.

Another study by Ong et al. (2014) in *Behavior Research and Therapy* examined the effects of Mindfulness-Based Stress Reduction (MBSR) on people with chronic insomnia. The results showed that mindfulness techniques helped participants break the cycle of anxiety and sleeplessness, leading to longer sleep duration and better overall rest.

Mindfulness practices also influence brain activity. In 2012, Dr. Gaëlle Desbordes at the Martinos Center for Biomedical Imaging, affiliated with the University of Massachusetts Medical School, conducted a study using functional magnetic resonance imaging (fMRI) to investigate the effects of mindfulness meditation on brain activity. The research revealed that participants who underwent an eight-week mindfulness-based stress reduction (MBSR) program exhibited reduced activity in the amygdala —a region of the brain associated with processing stress fear and emotions—even when they were not actively meditating. This finding suggests that mindfulness practices can lead to lasting changes in brain function, promoting a calmer response to stress.

Consider starting with a body scan meditation to incorporate mindfulness into your bedtime routine. This exercise involves lying comfortably and directing your attention to different body parts, releasing tension and fostering relaxation. Start by focusing on your toes, noticing any sensations or tension, and then gradually move your awareness up through your body, all the way to the top of your head. As you progress, allow yourself to let go of any tension or discomfort, embracing a sense of ease and relaxation. This practice helps you become more attuned to your body's needs and promotes a deep understanding of relaxation that can ease you into sleep.

Another effective mindfulness exercise is mindful breathing. Breathing is a natural rhythm we often take for granted, yet it holds the power to anchor our awareness and calm our minds. To practice mindful breathing, sit or lie down in a comfortable position and close your eyes. Focus your attention on the sensation of your breath as it enters and leaves your body. Notice the rise and fall of your chest, the coolness of the air as you inhale, and the warmth as you exhale. If your mind begins to wander, gently guide it back to the rhythm of your breath without judgment. This practice can be particularly helpful when your thoughts race at bedtime, providing a gentle focal point that encourages relaxation and presence.

Mindfulness has a substantial impact on stress reduction. Regular mindfulness practice has been shown to lower stress levels, improve emotional regulation, and enhance overall well-being. By cultivating a mindful approach to life, you can respond to stressors more calmly and clearly, reducing their impact on your sleep. Mindfulness encourages you to approach life's challenges with acceptance, allowing you to let go of the pressures that often keep you awake at night. This shift in mindset improves sleep quality and fosters a greater sense of peace and balance in your daily life.

7-Step Mindfulness Exercise for Better Sleep

This simple mindfulness routine can help you to quiet your mind and prepare your body for restful sleep. Practice it each night to create a calming bedtime ritual.

1. **Set the Environment:** Dim the lights, eliminate distractions, and find a comfortable position on your back with your arms resting at your sides. Close your eyes and take a moment to settle in.
2. **Focus on Your Breath:** Inhale slowly through your nose for a count of four, hold for a count of four, then exhale gently through your mouth for a count of six. Repeat this breathing pattern, letting each breath become slower and deeper.
3. **Body Scan Awareness:** Starting at the top of your head, bring your attention to each part of your body, moving down to your shoulders, arms, chest, and legs. Notice any areas of tension and allow them to relax with each exhale.

4. **Acknowledge and Release Thoughts:** As thoughts arise, acknowledge them without judgment. Imagine them floating away like clouds in the sky, gently bringing your focus back to your breath and body.

5. **Visualize Calmness:** Picture a peaceful scene, like waves gently lapping on the shore or a quiet forest. Imagine the sensations—cool air, soft sounds—and immerse yourself in the calmness of this mental space.

6. **Gratitude Reflection:** Silently reflect on three things you're grateful for from the day, no matter how small. This will shift your mind to a positive, peaceful state and reduce anxiety before sleep.

7. **Final Deep Breaths:** Take three final deep breaths, feeling your body grow heavier with each exhale. Allow yourself to drift into sleep, knowing that your mind and body are calm and ready for rest.

Consistency is key when it comes to reaping the long-term benefits of mindfulness. Like any skill, mindfulness requires regular practice to develop and sustain. Setting aside a specific time each day for mindfulness practice can help you to establish this habit and integrate it into your daily routine. Whether it's a few minutes in the morning, during lunch breaks, or as part of your bedtime ritual, finding a time that works for you is essential. Even dedicating just 10 minutes a day to mindfulness can bring about noticeable improvements in your sleep and overall well-being. Over time, this consistent practice can transform your relationship with sleep, leading to more restful nights and energized days.

Mindfulness Practice Journal

Consider keeping a mindfulness journal to track your experiences and progress:

- Record the time and duration of your mindfulness practice each day.
- Note any sensations, thoughts, or emotions that arise during your practice.
- Reflect on changes in sleep quality and stress levels over time.

This journaling exercise can enhance your mindfulness journey, providing insights and motivation to continue your practice. Embracing mindfulness opens the door to a more peaceful, restorative sleep experience, ultimately improving your productivity and well-being.

BREATHING EXERCISES TO INDUCE SLEEP

Breathing exercises hold a unique power to bring tranquility into your life, particularly when sleep seems elusive. The simple act of controlled breathing can activate the parasympathetic nervous system, often called the "rest and digest" system. Unlike its counterpart, the sympathetic nervous system, which is responsible for the "fight or flight" response, the parasympathetic system encourages relaxation and recovery. By engaging this system, you can effectively reduce your heart rate and lower blood pressure, creating an internal environment conducive to rest. These physiological changes prepare your body for sleep, acting like a natural sedative that gently calms the mind and body.

One of the most effective techniques in the realm of breathing exercises is the 4-7-8 method. This exercise is straightforward yet powerful. Begin by sitting or lying down comfortably. Inhale deeply through your nose for a count of four, feeling your chest and abdomen expand. Hold your breath for a count of seven, allowing the oxygen to circulate through your body. Finally, exhale slowly and completely through your mouth for a count of eight, letting go of any tension or stress with each breath. This rhythmic pattern works by slowing the heart rate and promoting relaxation. It is beneficial when your mind is racing at bedtime, as it shifts your focus to your breath, quieting mental chatter.

Another breathing technique worth exploring is alternate nostril breathing, known in yoga as Nadi Shodhana. This practice helps balance the brain's hemispheres and soothe the nervous system. Sit comfortably and close your right nostril with your right thumb to perform this exercise. Inhale deeply through your left nostril, then close it with your ring finger. Open your right nostril and exhale fully. Inhale through the right nostril, then close it and exhale through the left. Continue this alternating pattern for several cycles. This method calms the mind and enhances concentration and mental clarity, making it an excellent pre-sleep ritual to ease into relaxation.

Rhythmic breathing is crucial in signaling the body to relax and prepare for sleep. A steady breathing pattern serves as a metronome for your body, guiding it into a state of calmness and comfort. This predictability can be grounding, especially when anxiety or stress threatens to intrude upon your peace. By focusing on rhythmic breathing, you create a sense of stability that can override the chaos of a busy mind, allowing you to drift into sleep with greater ease.

Incorporating breathing exercises into your daily routine can be effortless and rewarding. You could practice while lying in bed, using the exercises as a gentle transition from wakefulness to sleep. Alternatively, consider integrating them into your evening wind-down routine after a warm bath or while listening to calming music. Again, the key is consistency; by making these exercises a regular part of your life, you reinforce a habit of relaxation that can transform your sleep quality. Experiment with different techniques to find what resonates most with you, and allow this practice to become a cherished part of your bedtime ritual.

PROGRESSIVE MUSCLE RELAXATION

Imagine a technique that gently guides you to shed the physical tension accumulated throughout the day, inviting your body to embrace a state of calm and ease. Progressive Muscle Relaxation (PMR) offers a simple yet powerful approach to reducing stress and enhancing sleep. At its core, PMR involves a cycle of tension and release, where you intentionally tense a muscle group and then relax it completely. This process fosters a deep sense of relaxation by heightening your awareness of physical sensations and encouraging the release of tension. By engaging different muscle groups deliberately, you teach your body to recognize and let go of stress, paving the way for a more restful sleep.

To practice PMR, find a comfortable position, either reclining in bed or sitting on a chair. Begin by focusing on your feet, curling your toes tightly, and holding that tension for a few seconds. As you release, allow the warmth of relaxation to spread through your feet. Next, move your attention to your calves, tensing and relaxing them. Continue this journey upwards, targeting each muscle group—thighs, abdomen, chest, arms, and finally, the face.

With each cycle, feel the weight of your worries melt away, replaced by a soothing calmness. This methodical progression helps to systematically eliminate tension, offering a clear path to tranquility that can ease you into sleep.

Practicing PMR has a remarkable psychological impact, particularly for those grappling with anxiety. By systematically releasing physical tension, PMR creates a ripple effect that extends to the mind, alleviating the burden of mental stress. As your body unwinds, so does your mind, fostering a sense of peace and safety that can counteract anxiety's grip. The practice teaches you to tune into your body's signals, promoting a deeper connection between your physical state and emotional well-being. This heightened awareness enhances relaxation and equips you with the tools to manage anxiety more effectively, leading to improved sleep quality and overall mental health.

Consistency is key to experiencing the full benefits of PMR. Just as regular exercise strengthens the body, consistent practice of PMR can fortify your ability to relax and manage stress. Aim to incorporate PMR into your daily routine, dedicating a few minutes each evening to this practice. Whether part of your bedtime ritual or a midday reset, regular engagement with PMR can yield cumulative effects, enhancing your resilience to stress over time. As you develop this habit, relaxation comes more naturally, allowing you to easily navigate life's challenges and sleep more soundly each night.

PMR Session Checklist

To help you get started with PMR, consider the following checklist:

- Find a quiet, comfortable space free from distractions.

- Work through your muscle groups from feet to head.
- Tense each muscle group for 5–10 seconds, then release for 15–20 seconds.
- Focus on the sensation of relaxation spreading through each muscle.
- Practice regularly for lasting benefits.

VISUALIZATION PRACTICES

Imagine a technique that can transform the chaotic whirl of thoughts in your mind into a serene landscape where calm and tranquility reign supreme. Visualization, a practice that taps into the power of mental imagery, offers precisely this result. By creating vivid mental pictures, you can guide your mind away from the day's stresses and toward a state of relaxation and readiness for sleep. Unlike other methods requiring physical involvement, visualization is an internal process that relies solely on your imagination. You can transport yourself to a place of peace and safety through guided imagery techniques, easing the transition from wakefulness to sleep.

Visualization is an effective stress reduction tool, offering a mental escape from the pressures that often accompany us to bed. By focusing on calming scenarios, you can diffuse the tension accumulated throughout the day. This redirection of thoughts helps lower stress levels, facilitating a more restful sleep experience. Visualization can be particularly beneficial for those who struggle with intrusive thoughts, as it provides a constructive method for shifting focus away from worries and onto more pleasant mental landscapes. In essence, visualization acts as a gentle guide, steering your mind toward a state of calm that nurtures both body and soul.

To harness the power of visualization, start by imagining a peaceful landscape. Picture yourself standing at the edge of a tranquil lake, the water so still it mirrors the sky above. The air is crisp and clean, carrying the faint scent of pine trees. As you breathe deeply, feel the cool earth beneath your feet, grounding you. Listen to the soft rustling of leaves whispering in the breeze. This vivid imagery calms your mind and engages your senses, creating a holistic experience that draws you into the present moment. Alternatively, you might visualize a calming journey, like taking a walk through a sunlit meadow or strolling along a quiet beach. Each step brings you closer to relaxation, allowing worries to drift away with the tide.

If you struggle with visualization, don't worry—like any skill, it can be developed with practice. Follow this step-by-step process to strengthen your ability to form mental images and use them for relaxation and sleep.

5-Step Process to Learn Visualization for Better Sleep

1. **Start with Simple Objects:** Begin by picturing everyday items you know, like an apple, a coffee mug, or your favorite chair. Close your eyes and try to see the shape, color, and texture in your mind. If the image feels unclear, focus on one detail, such as the shine on the apple or the curve of the mug's handle.
2. **Engage All Your Senses:** Instead of just "seeing" an image, try to feel, hear, and smell it. If you imagine a beach, think about the warmth of the sun, the scent of saltwater, and the sound of waves. Engaging multiple senses strengthens your brain's ability to create vivid mental scenes.
3. **Use Memory as a Guide:** If creating new images is difficult, recall a place or past experience. Think of a

childhood home, a vacation spot, or a favorite park. Remember as many details as possible—what you saw, heard, and felt in that moment.

4. **Describe What You Imagine:** If an image isn't clear, describe it to yourself as if you were telling a story. Say (silently or aloud), "The tree has rough bark, and the leaves move gently in the wind." This process reinforces visualization by engaging the language centers of your brain.

5. **Practice Guided Visualization:** Use an audiobook, guided meditation, or visualization script. As the narrator describes a scene, try to mentally paint the picture. Don't stress if you don't "see" things clearly at first—the goal is to immerse yourself in the feeling of the imagery, not just the visual details.

- **Bonus Tip—Keep Practicing:** Like any skill, visualization improves with daily practice. Spend 5–10 minutes each day using these techniques, and over time, your mental images will become sharper, making visualization an effective tool for relaxation and sleep.

The beauty of visualization lies in its adaptability. You can tailor your mental images to suit your personal preferences, ensuring that they resonate with your sense of peace and comfort. Some might find solace in the image of a cozy cabin nestled in the mountains. In contrast, others may prefer the gentle sway of a hammock beneath a canopy of stars. The key is to engage your creativity and personalize these scenarios, making them as vivid and compelling as possible. Doing so enhances their effectiveness, as your mind is more likely to engage with and respond to imagery that feels personally meaningful.

As you explore visualization, allow yourself to experiment and refine your practice. Consider which scenarios evoke the greatest sense of calm and relaxation, and then incorporate them into your nightly routine. Over time, visualization can become treasured ritual, a mental haven you visit each night to unwind and prepare for sleep. By embracing the power of your imagination, you can transform how you approach bedtime, paving the way for deeper, more restorative rest.

EVENING MEDITATION ROUTINES

Meditation is a gentle yet powerful practice that can prepare your mind and body for a peaceful night's sleep. By engaging in meditation before bed, you create a tranquil transition from the busyness of the day to the calm of nighttime rest. This practice offers more than just relaxation; it brings mental clarity, allowing your mind to release the clutter of thoughts and worries that often linger as you lay down. Meditation encourages focusing on the present, helping you clear your mind and create a serene space for sleep to unfold naturally. This mental clarity not only aids in falling asleep but also enhances the quality of your rest, leading to more refreshing mornings.

Creating a personalized meditation routine can be deeply rewarding, tailored to your unique needs and preferences. Start by selecting a meditation style that resonates with you. Some prefer guided meditations, where a soothing voice leads you through a series of calming visualizations or affirmations. Others might find solace in silent meditation, focusing on their breath or a mantra.

Exploring different meditation styles is important to see what feels most comfortable and effective. Once you've chosen your style, consider setting up a conducive environment that supports your practice. This might include dimming the lights, lighting a candle, or playing soft music to create a peaceful ambiance. A comfortable cushion or chair can also enhance your physical comfort, allowing you to fully engage in meditation without distractions.

Five Common Meditation Styles

Each of the follow methods cater to different needs and preferences.

1. **Mindfulness Meditation:** Focuses on being present in the moment, observing thoughts, feelings, and sensations without judgment. This style is rooted in Buddhist traditions and is often used for stress reduction and emotional regulation.

2. **Guided Visualization (or Guided Imagery):** Involves forming mental images of peaceful places or situations, often led by a teacher or recording. It engages the senses to promote relaxation and can be helpful for sleep and stress relief.

3. **Loving-Kindness Meditation:** Focuses on cultivating feelings of compassion, love, and kindness toward oneself and others. This style, known as Metta, is also a Buddhist practice. It can enhance emotional well-being and reduce negative emotions like anger and resentment.

4. **Body Scan Meditation:** Involves systematically focusing on different parts of the body, bringing awareness to sensations, tension, or discomfort. This practice is often used to promote relaxation and is a key part of Mindfulness-Based Stress Reduction (MBSR).

5. **Mantra Meditation:** Centers around the repetitive chanting or silent recitation of a word, phrase, or sound (such as "Om"). This repetition helps focus the mind, reduce distractions, and create a state of deep relaxation.

The power of meditation lies in its consistency. Like any habit, regular practice is key to reaping its full benefits. Aim to incorporate meditation into your nightly routine, dedicating a few minutes each evening to this practice. Over time, you'll likely find that regular meditation improves your sleep quality, helping you fall asleep more quickly and stay asleep longer. Consistency will strengthen your habit and deepen its impact as your mind and body become more attuned to the relaxation and clarity that meditation brings. The gradual accumulation of benefits that meditation offers can lead to significant improvements in both your sleep and overall well-being.

5 Simple Steps to Start Meditating for Beginners

If you're new to meditation, it can feel overwhelming at first—but it's simpler than you might think. Here's a step-by-step guide to help you get started and habituate yourself to consistent practice:

1. **Find a Quiet, Comfortable Space:** Choose a place where you won't be disturbed. Sit comfortably on a chair, cushion, or even lying down if that's easier. Keep your back straight but relaxed, and rest your hands on your lap or knees.
2. **Focus on Your Breath:** Close your eyes and bring your attention to your breathing. Notice the sensation of air entering and leaving your nose, the rise and fall of your chest, or the feeling of your belly expanding and contracting. Don't try to control your breath—just observe it.
3. **Notice When Your Mind Wanders:** It's natural for your mind to wander—that's part of the process! When you notice thoughts, distractions, or emotions popping up, gently bring your focus back to your breath without

judgment. Think of it like guiding a wandering puppy back to its path.

4. **Use a Focus Point (Optional):**

- If focusing on your breath feels difficult, try using a simple anchor:
- Repeat a calming word or phrase (like "peace" or "relax") silently in your mind.
- Focus on a sound, like soft background music or nature sounds.
- Visualize a peaceful image, like a candle flame or a calm ocean.

5. **End with Gratitude or Reflection:** When your timer goes off, take a few deep breaths before opening your eyes. Reflect on how you feel: lighter, calmer, or more aware. Even if the session felt challenging, acknowledge your effort and the time you gave yourself to slow down.

- **Bonus Tip:** Meditation isn't about "emptying your mind" or doing it perfectly. It's about showing up consistently, even just for a few minutes a day. The benefits grow over time as you build this habit.

To enhance your meditation experience, consider using meditation aids that can support and guide your practice. Guided meditation apps, available on your smartphone or tablet, offer a variety of sessions tailored to different needs and preferences. These apps provide structure and guidance, making maintaining focus and relaxation easier. Whether new to meditation or a seasoned practitioner, these tools can enrich your routine, offering new insights and techniques to explore. They can be particularly helpful on nights when your mind feels restless, providing a gentle anchor to return to the present moment.

As you settle into your meditation routine, remember that the process is as important as the outcome. Allow yourself to be present in each moment, embracing the practice with openness and curiosity. Over time, meditation can become a cherished part of your evening ritual, a time to unwind and reconnect with yourself before drifting into sleep. This practice enhances your sleep quality and fosters a deeper sense of peace and balance in your daily life, supporting your journey toward better rest and greater productivity.

As we conclude this chapter, I hope you've decided to try two or three of these powerful practices to help you with your sleep. These practices offer a pathway to tranquility, inviting you to embrace rest with open arms. As you integrate these techniques into your routine, you'll find that restful sleep is not just a distant goal but a tangible reality.

Summary:

- **Manage Sleep Anxiety** – Use cognitive reframing to shift from negative thoughts about sleep to positive ones. Try journaling to release worries before bed and practice self-compassion as you navigate sleep challenges.
- **Incorporate Mindfulness Practices** – Use techniques like body scans or mindful breathing to focus on the present moment, which will help you to reduce stress and pre-sleep anxiety. Regular mindfulness practice has been shown to improve sleep quality and reduce insomnia.
- **Practice Breathing Exercises** – Try the 4-7-8 method (inhale for 4 seconds, hold for 7, exhale for 8) or alternate

nostril breathing to activate the parasympathetic nervous system and promote relaxation before bed.

- **Use Progressive Muscle Relaxation (PMR)** – Systematically tense and release muscle groups from head to toe to reduce physical tension and calm the mind, helping you ease into sleep.
- **Experiment with Visualization Techniques** – Imagine peaceful, calming scenes (like a quiet beach or forest) to guide your mind away from stress and toward relaxation. Engage all your senses to make the imagery vivid and effective.
- **Create an Evening Meditation Routine** – Explore different styles like mindfulness meditation, guided visualization, or mantra meditation to calm your mind and prepare for restful sleep. Consistency is key to seeing long-term benefits.
- **Keep a Mindfulness Journal** – Track your progress with mindfulness and relaxation techniques, noting how they affect your sleep and stress levels. Reflecting on your practice can help identify what works best for you.

4

ESTABLISHING EFFECTIVE SLEEP HABITS

"A consistent bedtime isn't just for kids. Routine is the foundation of restful, restorative sleep."

— MATTHEW WALKER (NEUROSCIENTIST)

Crafting the perfect bedtime routine can feel like sculpting a masterpiece. Each person has unique needs and rhythms, which is why a one-size-fits-all approach doesn't work. Instead, consider your bedtime routine as a personal canvas, where each brushstroke—each activity—contributes to a picture of tranquility and rest. As you explore the elements that best support your journey to sleep, you'll find that consistency is your greatest ally. Establishing a structured routine signals to your body that it's time to wind down, much like dimming the lights before a grand performance. This signal is crucial for transitioning smoothly from the day's hustle to nighttime serenity.

Imagine the transition from day to night as a gentle descent into calmness. Start by incorporating activities that help bridge the gap between your active day and restful night. For many, reading a book offers a comforting escape—a chance to leave the day's worries behind and enter another world. Others might find solace in listening to calming music, letting each note wash over them like a soothing balm. Experiment with what resonates with you, and remember that these activities should be enjoyable, not a chore. A warm bath can further enhance this transition, as the increase in body temperature followed by a gradual cooling mimics the natural decline your body undergoes before sleep. This physiological change can help signal that it's time to rest, allowing you to glide toward sleep easily.

A journal can be a powerful tool for clearing your mind before bed. As thoughts swirl at the day's end, putting pen to paper can help free your mind from the clutter that might otherwise keep you awake. Consider jotting down the day's events, reflecting on moments of gratitude, or simply listing tomorrow's to-do list. This simple act of externalizing your thoughts can create mental space, reducing the mental chatter that often sabotages sleep. Additionally, journaling can serve as a ritual that signals the end of your day, providing closure and setting the stage for a restful night.

Time management is a crucial aspect of a successful bedtime routine. Allocating specific time slots for each activity ensures that your evening unfolds smoothly and without stress. Consider setting an alarm to remind yourself to start winding down, like a gentle nudge prompting you to begin your pre-sleep rituals. By structuring your evening, you create a predictable pattern that your body can rely on. This consistency helps regulate your internal clock, making it easier to fall asleep and wake up naturally.

Remember that change doesn't happen overnight. Gradual adjustments are key to establishing a sustainable routine that becomes a natural part of your life. If you aim to shift your bedtime, consider doing so in small increments, such as 15 minutes earlier each week. This approach allows your body to adapt without feeling forced, reducing resistance and increasing the likelihood of long-term success. As these changes take root, you'll likely notice improvements not just in how quickly you fall asleep but also in the quality of your rest. Embrace the process of trial and error, and be patient with yourself as you refine your routine.

Take a moment to reflect on your current bedtime routine. Which activities help you unwind, and which might be adding unnecessary stress? Jot down a few ideas for new activities to consider setting a realistic timeline for implementing these changes. Remember, it's about progress, not perfection.

Investing time and energy into crafting a personalized bedtime routine lays the foundation for more restful nights and productive days. This intentional approach to sleep can transform your evenings from chaotic to calming, allowing you to wake up refreshed and ready to tackle whatever comes your way.

THE 21-DAY HABIT FORMATION PLAN

The concept of habit formation is fascinating and practical, especially when considering its impact on sleep. The idea that you can reshape your behaviors and routines simply by repeating actions over a specific period is empowering. Historically, the notion that it takes 21 days to form a new habit comes from observations by Dr. Maxwell Maltz, who noticed his patients often took about three weeks to adjust to changes. Although modern research suggests the timeline can vary widely, typically taking anywhere from two to eight months depending on the individual and their behavior, the initial 21-day period remains a powerful starting point for many. This initial phase is crucial, acting as a foundation on which lasting habits are built.

Establishing new sleep habits can be broken down into a structured 21-day plan. Begin by identifying one or two specific changes you want to implement. Maybe it's going to bed at the same time every night or incorporating a relaxing activity before sleep. Use daily habit tracking sheets to monitor your progress. These sheets serve as visual reminders of your commitment and provide a clear record of your consistency. Set aside time for reflection and adjustment at the end of each week. Consider what worked, what didn't, and why. This reflective practice allows you to make informed tweaks to your routine, ensuring that each change is sustainable and effective.

Patience and persistence are your allies in this endeavor. It's easy to become discouraged when immediate results aren't apparent, especially when sleep is involved. However, remember that habit formation is a process, not an event. Consistency over time transforms a new behavior into an automatic part of your routine. Even when setbacks occur, and they will, it's essential to maintain your resolve. Each small step forward contributes to the bigger picture, gradually shifting your sleep patterns toward greater regularity and quality.

James Clear, author of *Atomic Habits*, says the following, "Habits are the compound interest of self-improvement. The effects of your habits multiply as you repeat them."

Motivation can wane over time, so it's helpful to employ strategies that keep your spirits high. Establishing achievable goals is a key tactic. Break your overarching objective into smaller, more manageable milestones. Celebrate each success, no matter how minor it may seem. Treat yourself to a relaxing activity or a favorite snack as a reward for hitting a weekly target. These rewards reinforce the positive changes you're making and provide a tangible incentive to continue. Another strategy is to visualize the benefits of improved sleep, such as increased energy or better mood, keeping these advantages at the forefront of your mind as you work through the challenges of habit formation.

Throughout this period, remember that you're not alone in your efforts. Sharing your goals with a friend or partner can offer additional support and accountability. Having someone to share your progress with can be incredibly motivating. Additionally, consider joining a community or forum in which others work on similar goals. The shared experiences and insights of others can provide valuable perspective and inspiration, helping you stay committed to your path.

Here are five notable platforms where participants focus on better sleep:

- **Pillow TalkTM by the National Sleep Foundation**: This online community allows members to share experiences and insights related to sleep and sleep disorders, fostering a supportive environment for those seeking to enhance their sleep quality.

americansleepmedicine.com

- **Sleepio**: Developed by sleep experts, Sleepio offers a digital sleep-improvement program featuring cognitive behavioral therapy (CBT) techniques. The platform includes an online community where users can discuss their progress and share tips for overcoming insomnia.

en.wikipedia.org/wiki/Sleepio

- **HealthUnlocked**: HealthUnlocked is a comprehensive health-focused social network that hosts various communities dedicated to sleep health. Members can connect with others facing similar challenges, exchange advice, and access resources to improve their sleep.

  en.wikipedia.org/wiki/HealthUnlocked

- **Reddit's r/Sleep**: This subreddit is a space where individuals discuss sleep-related topics, share personal experiences, and offer advice on improving sleep habits. The community covers various subjects, from sleep disorders to tips for better rest.
- **American Sleep Association Forums**: These forums provide a platform for discussing various sleep disorders and related treatments. Members can seek support, share experiences, and learn from others' journeys toward better sleep health.

Participating in these communities can provide practical advice, emotional support, and a connection with others striving for improved sleep.

Each day, as you mark your progress and reflect on your achievements, you'll find that the habits you once struggled to maintain begin to feel more natural. Your commitment to this 21-day plan is an investment in yourself that promises to yield benefits far beyond the immediate improvements in your sleep. As you build on these new habits, your changes will become more ingrained, providing a foundation for lasting sleep quality and overall well-being.

MANAGING SLEEP DEBT

Sleep debt is a term that captures the cumulative effect of insufficient sleep over time. It's akin to a financial debt, where each missed hour of sleep adds up, eventually leading to significant consequences for your physical and mental health. This often manifests as persistent fatigue, making it difficult to concentrate and perform daily tasks. You might find yourself snapping at loved ones over minor irritations, unable to muster the patience you once had. These symptoms of fatigue and irritability disrupt your personal life and professional environment, impacting productivity and decision-making capabilities. If you're like me, you may come down with a cold or the flu. Over time, chronic sleep debt can lead to more severe health issues, such as increased risks of hypertension, diabetes, and even heart disease.

A strategy focused on recovery will mitigate the effects of sleep debt. Scheduled catch-up sleep sessions can be an effective way to repay this debt gradually and involve setting aside specific times to sleep longer than usual, perhaps during weekends. By allowing your body to rest more deeply, you begin to restore the balance disrupted by previous sleep deprivation. However, be mindful not to oversleep, which could disrupt your natural sleep cycle further. Instead, aim for consistency, gradually increasing your sleep duration in manageable increments. Prioritizing sleep during weekends is another practical approach. Using these days to catch up, you create a buffer that helps compensate for lost sleep during the week. It's a delicate balance, but with thoughtful planning, you can start alleviating the burden of sleep debt.

Addressing the root causes of sleep debt is pivotal for long-term improvement. Often, stress and anxiety are culprits that prevent you from getting the rest you need. Implementing stress management techniques can be transformative. It's also beneficial to critically assess other contributing factors, such as workload or lifestyle choices, and make necessary adjustments. Identifying what's keeping you awake allows you to tackle sleep deprivation at its source, reducing the need for catch-up sleep in the future.

Preventing sleep debt from accumulating at a later time requires a proactive approach. Regular sleep audits can be incredibly helpful here. You gain insight into what works and needs adjustment by periodically reviewing your sleep patterns and habits. This reflection can guide you in maintaining a healthy sleep schedule that accommodates your lifestyle and your body's needs. Consider setting reminders or alarms to signal when it's time to start winding down for the night. These small cues can differentiate between staying up too late and getting your needed rest. Engaging in these preventative measures not only helps avoid sleep debt but also enhances your overall quality of life, allowing you to function at your best.

THE ART OF NAPPING

Imagine a world where a brief afternoon nap could recharge your brain and boost your mood without disrupting your night's sleep. When done strategically, napping offers many benefits that can enhance your daily performance. A well-timed nap can increase alertness, improve cognitive function, and elevate your mood. It's a quick reset button for your brain, helping you tackle the second half of your day with renewed energy and focus. Contrary to the misconception that napping interferes with nighttime sleep, an adequately timed nap can complement your sleep routine, allowing you to feel more rested and alert.

Napping is more than just a quick rest—it's a scientifically proven tool to enhance cognitive performance, mood, and overall health.

Research shows that short naps can restore alertness, improve memory, and even reduce the risk of chronic diseases.

A landmark study by NASA (2008) on astronauts and pilots revealed that a 26-minute nap improved performance by 34% and alertness by 54%. This highlights how even brief rest periods can dramatically enhance focus and efficiency, making naps particularly valuable for those with demanding schedules.

Another study from Harvard Medical School (2002) found that napping helps consolidate declarative memory—the ability to recall facts and knowledge. Participants who took a 60–90-minute nap showed significant improvement in learning and recall tasks compared to those who remained awake.

Naps also regulate emotions. A study published in *The Journal of Clinical Endocrinology & Metabolism* (2015) found that short naps can reduce stress and counteract the negative hormonal effects of sleep deprivation, such as increased cortisol levels.

The ideal nap length varies depending on the desired benefits; 10–20-minute naps offer quick boosts in alertness without grogginess, while 60–90-minute naps allow for a full sleep cycle, enhancing creativity and problem-solving. However, naps longer than 30 minutes can lead to sleep inertia—temporary grogginess after waking.

Incorporating naps into your routine, especially when nighttime sleep is insufficient, can improve mental clarity, emotional balance, and physical health. Backed by science, napping is a powerful, natural tool to optimize daily performance and long-term well-being.

To reap these benefits, it's crucial to understand the guidelines for effective napping. Timing is everything. The ideal nap occurs in the early afternoon—typically after lunch when energy levels naturally dip. This timing aligns with your body's natural circadian rhythms, making it easier to fall asleep quickly and wake up refreshed. I suggest you aim for a nap length of 20–30 minutes. This duration is long enough to enhance alertness without entering the deeper stages of sleep. Your environment also plays a role; a cool, quiet, dark space can help you fall asleep faster and enjoy a more restful nap.

If you're looking for a brief respite, a power nap is your best bet. Longer naps can be beneficial for more substantial rest, but they require careful planning to avoid interfering with your nighttime sleep.

Despite the clear advantages, napping is often misunderstood. A common myth suggests that napping is only for the lazy, but science tells a different story. By understanding how naps fit into your overall sleep strategy, you can use them to your advantage.

CONSISTENCY IN SLEEP SCHEDULES

Imagine waking up each morning feeling refreshed, with your body naturally attuned to the rhythm of the day. This harmony is often disrupted by irregular sleep schedules, confusing your internal clock and making restful sleep elusive. A consistent sleep-wake schedule acts as a gentle guide, aligning your body's circadian rhythms with the natural light-dark cycle. This synchronization reduces sleep latency, the time it takes to fall asleep, allowing you to drift off more easily. Your body thrives on routine, and adhering to regular bedtimes and wake-up times reinforces this, signaling that it's time to rest and rejuvenate.

Practical strategies can be invaluable for maintaining consistency in your sleep schedule. Begin by setting an alarm not just for waking up but also for bedtime. This reminder prompts you to start winding down, helping you stick to your chosen schedule. While it's tempting to sleep in on a day away from work, try to wake up within an hour of your usual time to prevent disrupting your internal clock.

Social and work commitments often challenge our best-laid sleep plans. Late-night events, early meetings, and unpredictable schedules can throw a wrench into your routine. Planning social activities around your sleep schedule might require creativity but can make a significant difference. Consider meeting friends for brunch rather than a late dinner or carve out time for important tasks earlier in the day. Communicate your sleep goals to those around you, enlisting their support and understanding. This collaboration can help reduce conflict between your social life and your need for rest, allowing you to enjoy both without sacrificing your well-being.

Flexibility within your schedule can also prevent unnecessary stress. Life rarely adheres to a perfect plan, and occasional deviations from your routine are normal. Allow yourself the grace to adjust when necessary, recognizing that perfection isn't the goal. A dinner that runs late or an early morning meeting doesn't have to derail your entire schedule. By building in a bit of flexibility, you balance routine with spontaneity. On weekends, for instance, minor deviations can be a treat rather than a setback as long as they remain the exception rather than the rule.

Consider the delicate balance between routine and flexibility as a dance. Whether firm or fluid, each step contributes to a rhythm that supports your health and productivity. Establishing regular sleep patterns isn't about rigid adherence to rules but about understanding and responding to your body's needs with kindness and consistency. By prioritizing a schedule that respects your natural rhythms, you create an environment where sleep comes naturally and effortlessly, night after night.

AVOIDING COMMON SLEEP PITFALLS

In the quest for a good night's sleep, it's easy to overlook everyday habits that quietly sabotage our rest. As I've talked about, one of the most insidious culprits is late-night screen use. Not only does the blue light emitted from phones, tablets, and computers mimic daylight, but scrolling through social media or watching videos right before bed can also stimulate your mind, keeping you mentally active when your body craves rest. It's a modern dilemma where the convenience of technology clashes with the natural rhythms of sleep.

Caffeine, our faithful companion in combating afternoon slumps, can wreak havoc on sleep if consumed too late in the day. While it can provide a much-needed boost, caffeine remains in the system for several hours, potentially interfering with your ability to fall asleep. The afternoon cup of coffee or evening chocolate dessert might seem harmless, but they can contribute to restless nights. Understanding the half-life of caffeine and timing your consumption can significantly impact your sleep quality. Limiting caffeine intake to mornings or early afternoons can help ensure it doesn't disrupt your nighttime rest.

Recognizing and rectifying these pitfalls requires a conscious effort. Start by setting a technology curfew and establish a caffeine curfew. Setting a specific time in the afternoon as your cutoff allows your body ample time to process the caffeine before bedtime. These minor adjustments can create a more sleep-friendly environment, paving the way for restful nights.

Lifestyle choices extend beyond screen time and caffeine, influencing sleep more subtly. A balanced diet rich in nutrients can support the sleep cycle. At the same time, regular physical activity helps regulate energy levels and reduces stress. However, timing is key. Engaging in vigorous exercise too close to bedtime can leave you wired rather than tired. Aim to finish workouts at least a few hours before bed to give your body time to cool down. Stress management also plays a critical role. Daily stressors can accumulate, leading to a racing mind at night. As I've talked about, incorporating relaxation techniques can help calm your nervous system, making it easier to drift into sleep.

Self-awareness is your greatest tool in identifying personal sleep pitfalls.

As you become more attuned to the factors that influence your sleep, you'll find that small changes can lead to significant improvements. You create a foundation for more restful nights and energized days by avoiding common pitfalls and embracing healthier habits. With a clearer understanding of your sleep patterns and triggers, you're better equipped to make choices that support your overall well-being.

Summary:

- **Create a Consistent Bedtime Routine** – Engage in relaxing activities like reading, journaling, or taking a warm bath to signal your body that it's time to wind down. Stick to a consistent bedtime and wake-up time, even on weekends.
- **Follow the 21-Day Habit Formation Plan** – Introduce new sleep habits gradually over 21 days. Track your progress with habit sheets, adjust as needed, and celebrate small milestones to build lasting routines.

- **Manage Sleep Debt Strategically** – Catch up on missed sleep with extra rest on weekends or by going to bed earlier, but avoid oversleeping to prevent disrupting your circadian rhythm.
- **Incorporate Power Naps Wisely** – Take short naps (10–20 minutes) in the early afternoon to boost alertness without affecting nighttime sleep. If needed, use longer naps (60–90 minutes) for a complete sleep cycle and cognitive restoration.
- **Avoid Common Sleep Pitfalls** – Limit caffeine after early afternoon, avoid screens an hour before bed, and finish intense workouts at least three hours before bedtime to prevent overstimulation.
- **Optimize Your Sleep Schedule Flexibly** – Set reminders for bedtime and adjust your routine gradually if you shift your sleep times. Allow occasional flexibility, but aim for regular sleep patterns overall.

5

ADDRESSING SPECIFIC SLEEP CHALLENGES

"When you can't sleep, it's not about trying harder, it's about letting go."

— ECKHART TOLLE (*AUTHOR OF THE POWER OF NOW*)

SLEEP LATENCY

Imagine lying in bed, the room dark and quiet, yet your mind races with thoughts, refusing to quiet down. The clock continues to tick, each minute amplifying the frustration. This experience, known as sleep latency, refers to the time it takes to transition from wakefulness to sleep. For many adults, prolonged sleep latency is a nightly struggle, exacerbated by pre-sleep anxiety and irregular sleep schedules. Pre-sleep anxiety often stems from the demands of daily life, with worries about work, relationships, or personal challenges bubbling to the surface just as you hope to relax. These anxious thoughts create a mental whirlwind, making it difficult to drift into slumber. Similarly, irregular sleep schedules can disrupt your internal clock, leading to sleep onset inconsistencies and perpetuating the sleeplessness cycle.

Addressing sleep latency requires a multifaceted approach, where cognitive-behavioral strategies are pivotal. Cognitive behavioral therapy for insomnia (CBT-I) is a well-documented strategy that can significantly reduce sleep latency by altering the thought patterns that delay sleep. Cognitive restructuring, a key component of CBT-I, involves identifying and challenging negative beliefs about sleep. For instance, if you often think, "I'll never fall asleep," you might reframe this to, "I've had restful nights before, and I can again." By transforming these thoughts, you create a more conducive mental environment for sleep, reducing anxiety, and improving sleep onset.

Sleep Latency Improvement Checklist

Consider incorporating these changes to your routine to improve sleep latency:

- Practice cognitive restructuring to challenge negative sleep thoughts.
- Engage in progressive relaxation exercises focused on breathing.
- Explore guided visualization of peaceful scenarios to calm the mind.
- Reduce evening screen time to support natural melatonin production.
- Establish a calming pre-sleep wind-down period with relaxing activities.

Addressing the mental and physical barriers to sleep creates an environment where restful nights become more attainable. These strategies can transform your approach to sleep, fostering quicker sleep onset and more rejuvenating rest.

STAYING ASLEEP ALL NIGHT

Waking up in the middle of the night can be frustrating, and many face this issue without understanding why. Several factors can disrupt sleep continuity, leaving you groggy and unrested by morning. Stress and anxiety are the primary culprits. Often, unresolved worries or even subconscious stressors cause our brains to remain active, ready to wake us at the slightest provocation. These mental disturbances can easily pull you out of deep sleep, leaving you staring at the ceiling instead of dreaming peacefully.

Beyond mental factors, physical disturbances in your environment play a significant role. Noise from a passing car, a neighbor's late-night activities, or even the hum of an appliance can jolt you awake. Similarly, room temperature, whether too hot or cold, can disrupt your sleep cycles as your body struggles to find comfort.

Practical interventions can be quite effective in minimizing these disruptions. White noise machines are a popular solution for masking sudden or persistent noise. Whether it's the sound of a gentle rain or consistent static, these machines can help drown out disturbances that might otherwise wake you.

Understanding sleep cycles offers insight into why we wake at night and how we can manage these awakenings. Sleep occurs in cycles, typically lasting about 90 minutes, rotating between different stages, including light sleep, deep sleep, and REM sleep. Most awakenings tend to occur during lighter sleep stages when the body is closer to wakefulness. By aligning your sleep schedule to fit these natural cycles, you can improve your chances of waking up at the end of a sleep cycle rather than in the middle.

This can leave you feeling more refreshed and less disoriented. It's helpful to time your bedtime and wake-up time to coincide with completing a full cycle, allowing your body to transition to wakefulness more smoothly.

Even with precautions, awakenings can still happen, and having strategies to return to sleep quickly is essential. Many people experience nighttime awakenings, but understanding the causes and having strategies to address them can make a world of difference. By minimizing disruptions and employing techniques to ease back into sleep, you create an environment conducive to uninterrupted rest.

GETTING BACK TO SLEEP

Falling back asleep can feel frustrating and elusive. Whether it's due to stress, environmental factors, or disruptions in your sleep cycle, waking up doesn't have to ruin your night. Scientific research offers practical strategies to help you return to restful sleep quickly and naturally.

The first step is to stay calm. It's natural to wake up briefly at night, but stressing about it can make it harder to drift back to sleep. Avoid checking the time, as this can trigger sleep performance anxiety, making you feel pressured to fall asleep quickly. A study in *Behavior Research and Therapy* (2002) showed that focusing on the clock increases stress hormones like cortisol, which keeps you awake longer. Turn your clock away or place your phone out of reach to avoid temptation.

Of course, you can employ any of the techniques I've mentioned to calm down and fall asleep.

DEALING WITH NIGHTMARES

Nightmares can be more than just unsettling dreams; they are vivid experiences that can leave your heart racing and your mind on edge, disrupting your sleep and impacting your mood well into the next day. At their core, nightmares often arise from a mix of psychological and physiological factors. Stress is a major contributor, with anxiety and tension from daily life spilling over into our subconscious, manifesting as distressing dreams. When our minds are burdened with unresolved stressors, the result can be a restless night punctuated by vivid and troubling images.

Medication side effects can also play a role, with certain drugs known to alter dream patterns and increase the frequency of nightmares. These medications can disrupt the natural sleep architecture, leading to more intense and memorable dreams. Check on any prescriptions you may take for side effects around sleep.

One effective method for reducing nightmare frequency is imagery rehearsal therapy (IRT). A study by Krakow et al. (2001) in *The Journal of the American Medical Association* found that IRT significantly reduced nightmares and improved overall sleep quality in PTSD patients. This cognitive-behavioral technique involves visualizing a recurring nightmare and consciously altering its storyline to create a more positive outcome. You can retrain your brain to diminish the nightmare's power by rehearsing this new version during waking hours. By changing the narrative of disturbing dreams, IRT helps decrease nighttime awakenings and fosters deeper, more restorative sleep.

Stress management practices are equally important. Incorporating relaxation techniques such as yoga or meditation into your daily routine can help lower overall stress levels, reducing the likelihood of stress-induced nightmares. Regular physical activity is another powerful strategy, as exercise releases endorphins, which naturally combat stress and promote better sleep.

When nightmares do occur, the moments on waking can be fraught with anxiety. It's crucial to have strategies to calm your mind and body, allowing you to return to sleep. Calming breathing exercises can be particularly effective. Focusing on slow, deep breaths can activate the parasympathetic nervous system, which helps reduce the body's stress response. Reassuring self-talk is another tool to help ease your transition back to sleep. Remind yourself that the nightmare is just a creation of your mind and holds no real power over you. This mental reassurance can help dissipate lingering fear and anxiety, paving the way for a return to restful slumber.

Lifestyle factors, including diet, can also influence the intensity and frequency of nightmares. Heavy meals before bed can lead to indigestion and discomfort, disrupting sleep and provoking unsettling dreams. The digestion process requires energy and increases body temperature, which can interfere with the natural cooling and relaxation processes needed for deep sleep. To minimize the risk of nightmares, aim to have your last meal at least two to three hours before bedtime. Opt for light, easily digestible snacks, such as a small bowl of yogurt or a handful of almonds, if you're feeling peckish in the evening. Additionally, reducing your intake of caffeine and alcohol, especially in the hours leading up to sleep, can further support a more peaceful night.

By understanding the origins of nightmares and implementing strategies to mitigate their impact, you can transform your nights into a period of rejuvenation rather than restlessness. Addressing both the psychological and lifestyle factors that contribute to nightmares may not eradicate them, yet actively recognizing these triggers can significantly reduce the frequency and severity of unpleasant sleep disruptions.

MANAGING SLEEP APNEA NATURALLY

Sleep apnea is a condition that significantly disrupts sleep quality and overall health. It occurs when breathing repeatedly stops and starts during sleep. You might recognize it by its hallmark symptoms: loud snoring and moments of gasping for air. These breathing interruptions can last a few seconds to minutes, jolting you awake and preventing deep, restorative sleep. As a result, many people with sleep apnea experience chronic daytime fatigue, which can impair daily functioning and increase the risk of accidents. This persistent tiredness stems from the brain and body not getting enough oxygen at night, which affects your energy levels and concentration.

Specific lifestyle changes are beneficial to mitigate sleep apnea symptoms. Managing weight through a balanced diet and regular exercise can substantially impact your body's resilience to the causes of sleep apnea. Excess weight, particularly around the neck, can constrict airways, exacerbating apnea symptoms. Exercise not only aids in weight management but also strengthens respiratory muscles, improving breathing efficiency. Side sleeping positions can also help. Sleeping on your back may cause the tongue and soft tissues to fall back, blocking the airway. By shifting to your side, you can clear air passages, reducing the frequency and severity of apnea events.

In addition to these changes, breathing exercises and devices can further enhance airway function during sleep. Positional therapy devices, such as specialized pillows or wearable gadgets, encourage side sleeping and maintain optimal head and neck alignment.

These devices can gently nudge you to the side if you roll onto your back, ensuring that airways remain open.

Incorporating breathing exercises into your routine can also be beneficial. Techniques such as diaphragmatic breathing (the 4-7-8 method described earlier) can increase lung capacity and improve overall breathing patterns. Practicing these exercises regularly can strengthen the muscles involved in respiration, potentially reducing apnea episodes.

Seeking Further Help for Sleep Apnea

There are times when lifestyle changes and non-invasive methods may not be enough to help you overcome sleeping and nighttime breathing difficulties. If you continue to experience persistent symptoms despite implementing the strategies above, then it may be time to seek professional help.

Consulting with a healthcare provider is crucial if you notice signs like loud snoring, chronic daytime sleepiness, or frequent awakenings with gasping. A sleep study can diagnose the severity of your condition and determine the most appropriate treatment. Medical interventions, such as continuous positive airway pressure (CPAP) machines, might be recommended for moderate to severe cases. These devices keep airways open by providing a steady stream of air through a mask, significantly improving sleep quality and reducing health risks associated with untreated sleep apnea.

Recognizing when to seek help is vital in managing sleep apnea effectively, ensuring you achieve the restful, uninterrupted sleep your body needs for optimal health and performance.

TRAVEL AND SLEEP

Sleep Better on an Airplane

Sleeping on an airplane, whether in the tight quarters of a coach or the relative luxury of business class, presents unique challenges. The combination of cabin noise, fluctuating temperatures, cramped seating, and general discomfort can make restful in-flight sleep seem impossible. However, by preparing before your flight, optimizing your environment, and using proven relaxation techniques, you can significantly improve the quality of your rest and arrive at your destination feeling refreshed.

Dressing comfortably in loose, breathable layers can help regulate your body temperature, which is often difficult to control in the fluctuating environment of an airplane cabin. Once onboard, creating a sleep-conducive environment is essential, especially in coach where space is limited. Seat selection plays a critical role— window seats offer something to lean against and prevent interruptions from seatmates needing to get up. Choosing a spot near the front of the plane reduces exposure to engine noise and turbulence while avoiding seats near bathrooms or galleys minimizes disturbances from passenger traffic.

Travel accessories can further enhance comfort. A high-quality neck pillow supports and reduces neck strain, while an eye mask blocks out cabin lights and glowing screens from nearby passengers. Noise-canceling headphones or simple earplugs help drown out ambient sounds, promoting deeper sleep. Harvard Medical School research emphasizes the importance of reducing noise to achieve more restorative rest. Even small adjustments, like reclining your seat slightly or using a rolled-up blanket for lower back support, can significantly affect comfort and sleep quality.

In business class, where amenities are more generous, there are still ways to enhance your sleep experience. Lie-flat seats offer a huge advantage, but adjusting them to align your hips and spine can prevent discomfort and promote better rest. Airlines often provide blankets, pillows, and amenity kits in business class, and layering these comfort items for warmth and support can further optimize your sleeping posture. Although business-class cabins offer better lighting options, bringing your own eye mask ensures complete darkness.

In 2011, a study published in the *Journal of Clinical Endocrinology & Metabolism* examined the impact of room light exposure before bedtime on melatonin production. The researchers found that exposure to standard indoor lighting (<200 lux) during the evening significantly suppressed melatonin levels in 99% of the participants, delaying its onset and shortening its duration by approximately 90 minutes compared to dim light conditions (<3 lux). Additionally, exposure to room light during usual sleep hours reduced melatonin levels by more than 50% in most cases. These findings suggest that typical indoor lighting in the evening can drastically disrupt melatonin signaling, potentially affecting sleep quality and other physiological processes regulated by melatonin.

Other studies show similar results and underscore the importance of minimizing light exposure before and during sleep to maintain optimal melatonin production and support healthy sleep patterns whether on a plane or at home in your bedroom.

Regardless of your seating class, what you consume during your flight plays a crucial role in how well you sleep. While alcohol may initially make you feel drowsy, it significantly disrupts the sleep cycle and especially reduces REM sleep, the necessary stage for emotional regulation and memory consolidation. In a 2013 study published in *Alcoholism: Clinical and Experimental Research*, alcohol consumption before bed led to fragmented sleep and frequent awakenings, making it harder to achieve restorative rest. Since alcohol induces shallow sleep prone to interruptions, it's best to avoid it before and during your flight in order to experience deeper, uninterrupted rest.

Avoiding heavy meals is also critical, as a full stomach and active digestion can disrupt sleep cycles. Opt for light meals and avoid caffeine several hours before sleep to further reduce the risk of sleep disturbances. Staying hydrated is equally important, as airplane cabins are notoriously dry. Drinking water throughout your flight helps prevent dehydration. It's also wise to moderate intake close to slumber to avoid frequent bathroom trips.

If you find it difficult to relax, incorporating the techniques in this book will help you relax and fall asleep. While airplane sleep might never be as restful as sleeping at home, thoughtful preparation and minor adjustments can make a significant difference. By implementing these tips, you can arrive at your destination feeling more refreshed and energized to make the most of your trip.

Handling Jet Lag and Shift Work

Traveling across time zones or working non-traditional hours can significantly disrupt your body's natural rhythms, which affects natural regulation of your sleep-wake cycles, hormones, and bodily functions. Rapid travel across multiple time zones causes your internal clock to be out of sync with the new local time. This misalignment can lead to symptoms like fatigue, insomnia, and difficulty concentrating. Similarly, shift work forces your body to operate outside its preferred rhythm, leading to chronic sleep deprivation and a host of related health issues.

To minimize the effects of jet lag, gradual schedule adjustments before travel can be remarkably effective. As your trip approaches, start shifting your sleep schedule by an hour or two toward that of the destination time zone. This helps ease your body into its new rhythm gradually, reducing the shock of sudden change.

Since I travel internationally relatively often, I can share one of my personal tricks with you. Upon arrival at my destination, I take on the current zone right away and go to bed at the bedtime of my new time zone. For example, when I arrive in Europe at midday or in the morning, I force myself to stay up until ten or eleven at night. This way, I'm exhausted and won't have trouble falling asleep, and I usually stay asleep for most of the night. Given this timing strategy, I also try to book a flight that arrives around midday or early afternoon.

Light exposure management is another powerful tool. Light is a primary cue for setting your circadian rhythm, so seeking natural sunlight during the day and minimizing exposure to artificial light at night can help reset your internal clock. If natural light isn't accessible, consider using a light therapy box to simulate daylight. This can be especially helpful for aligning your sleep schedule with the new time zone.

Shift workers face a unique challenge, as their work hours often conflict with natural circadian rhythms. Creating a consistent sleep environment is crucial. Darkening your bedroom with blackout curtains and using white noise machines can help simulate nighttime, encouraging better sleep during daylight hours. Establishing a regular sleep schedule, even on days off, supports your body's adaptation to irregular hours. Strategic nap planning can also alleviate fatigue. Short naps during breaks or before a shift can provide a quick energy boost without interfering with nighttime sleep. Keep naps to 20-30 minutes to avoid entering deep sleep.

Maintaining a healthy lifestyle is essential in coping with the challenges of jet lag and shift work. Avoid heavy meals close to bedtime, as they can interfere with sleep. Regular physical activity is equally important, as it helps regulate your sleep-wake cycle and reduces stress. Even short bursts of exercise, like a brisk walk, can boost your mood and energy levels. Managing stress through relaxation techniques such as mindfulness or yoga can improve sleep quality, helping you feel refreshed despite irregular hours.

Jet lag and shift work are inevitable parts of life for many, but understanding their impact allows you to take proactive steps to mitigate these effects. By aligning your habits with your body's natural rhythms as much as possible, you can improve your sleep quality and overall well-being, even in challenging circumstances.

SEXUAL ACTIVITY AND YOUR SLEEP

Sex with a partner or on your own is often touted as a natural sleep aid, and scientific research supports this connection. Engaging in sexual activity can promote relaxation, reduce stress, and improve sleep quality due to hormonal shifts and the release of feel-good chemicals in the brain. Understanding the physiological mechanisms behind this activity can help individuals harness sexual activity as part of a healthy bedtime routine.

During sexual activity, the body releases a cocktail of hormones that contribute to feelings of relaxation and sleepiness. One of the primary hormones involved is oxytocin, often called the "love hormone." Oxytocin is released during intimate physical contact, including sex and masturbation, fostering feelings of connection and calm. A study published in *Frontiers in Public Health* (2017) found that higher oxytocin levels are associated with reduced stress and increased feelings of relaxation, both of which are conducive to sleep.

In addition to oxytocin, sexual activity leads to the release of prolactin, a hormone linked to satisfaction and relaxation. Prolactin levels rise significantly after orgasm, and this spike is closely associated with the feeling of drowsiness that many people experience post-sex. Research published in the *Journal of Sexual Medicine* (2006) found that prolactin levels were 400% higher after orgasm, particularly in men, suggesting a strong connection between sexual release and the body's readiness for sleep.

Organisms also help reduce levels of cortisol, the body's primary stress hormone. Elevated cortisol levels can interfere with the body's natural sleep cycles, particularly by disrupting REM sleep, the stage associated with dreaming and cognitive restoration. A study from the University of Michigan (2019) highlighted how orgasm reduces cortisol levels, thereby decreasing stress and facilitating the body's transition into restful sleep.

For men and women alike, the post-orgasmic release of endorphins—the body's natural painkillers and mood boosters—contributes to well-being and relaxation. Endorphins can help alleviate mild physical discomfort or restlessness, both of which might otherwise hinder the ability to fall asleep. Moreover, sexual activity increases the parasympathetic nervous system's response, which promotes calm and recovery, further enhancing the body's readiness for sleep.

While much of the research has historically focused on men, recent studies indicate that women experience similar sleep benefits from sexual activity. A 2019 study published in *Sleep Health* surveyed over 800 participants and found that both men and women reported improved sleep quality following orgasm, regardless of whether it was achieved through partnered sex or on their own.

However, it's important to note that the impact of sexual activity on sleep can vary depending on the individual and the context. For some, particularly those who associate sex with emotional stress or anxiety, sexual activity might not have the same relaxing effect. Additionally, vigorous activity close to bedtime can temporarily raise heart rate and body temperature, which could delay sleep onset for some individuals. In such cases, allowing time to wind down post-activity can help mitigate these effects.

Integrating sexual activity into a bedtime routine—whether for stress relief, relaxation, or simply as part of a healthy lifestyle—can contribute to better sleep quality and overall well-being. As with any sleep strategy, the key is understanding what works best for you and creating a personalized routine that aligns with your body's unique needs.

COPING WITH SLEEP PARALYSIS

Sleep paralysis is a phenomenon that can be both terrifying and bewildering. Picture this: You find yourself awake yet unable to move or speak as if trapped between the realm of sleep and consciousness. It often feels like an invisible weight is pressing down on you, rendering you immobile and vulnerable. This condition occurs when the transition between wakefulness and sleep is disrupted, leaving you partially aware but unable to act. Common triggers include inconsistent sleep patterns, stress, and chronic sleep deprivation. When your sleep schedule is erratic, your body struggles to maintain the delicate balance needed for seamless transitions between sleep stages. Stress, too, plays a significant role, as it can disrupt sleep architecture and increase the likelihood of sleep paralysis episodes.

Managing sleep paralysis involves fostering a regular sleep routine. Maintaining consistent sleep and wake times helps your body establish a stable rhythm, reducing the chances of experiencing these unsettling events. Consider creating a bedtime ritual that encourages relaxation and signals to your body that it's time to wind down, as I've been writing about. By reinforcing your body's internal clock, you can minimize the disruptions that lead to sleep paralysis.

Beyond routine, addressing the fear associated with sleep paralysis is crucial. The experience can be frightening, leaving you anxious about future episodes. Cognitive behavioral therapy (CBT) techniques offer effective tools for managing this fear. CBT can help you reframe negative thoughts associated with sleep paralysis, replacing them with more constructive beliefs. For instance, understanding that sleep paralysis is a temporary and harmless state can alleviate some of your anxiety. Mindfulness practices also play a role in reducing fear. By cultivating a present-focused mindset, you can learn to observe the sensations of sleep paralysis without judgment or panic. Mindfulness encourages acceptance, helping you remain calm during episodes and reducing the overall stress response.

4 Key Steps in Cognitive Behavioral Therapy for Insomnia (CBT-I):

1. **Identify Negative Sleep Thoughts:** Recognize and write down unhelpful thoughts or beliefs about sleep, such as "I'll never fall asleep" or "If I don't sleep, tomorrow will be a disaster."
2. **Challenge and Reframe These Thoughts:** Examine the evidence for and against these beliefs. Replace them with more balanced, realistic thoughts, like "Even if I don't sleep perfectly, I can still get through the day."

3. **Practice Stimulus Control:** Limit your bed's association with wakefulness. Only go to bed when you're sleepy, and if you can't fall asleep within 20 minutes, get up and do a quiet activity until you feel tired again.
4. **Incorporate Relaxation Techniques:** Use methods like deep breathing, progressive muscle relaxation, or mindfulness meditation to calm your mind and body before bed. This will reduce anxiety and promote restful sleep.

While self-management strategies can be effective, there may be times when professional help is warranted. If sleep paralysis episodes persist or severely impact your quality of life, consulting a specialist is advisable. A healthcare provider can assess your symptoms, rule out underlying sleep disorders, and recommend tailored treatments. In some cases, medication or therapy may be necessary to address the root causes of sleep disturbances.

As you navigate the complexities of sleep paralysis, remember that you are not alone. Many individuals experience this condition, and with the right strategies, you can reduce its frequency and impact. By prioritizing sleep routine regularity, addressing associated fears, and seeking professional guidance when needed, you can reclaim control over your sleep and enhance your overall well-being.

Summary:

- **Reduce Sleep Latency** – Implement cognitive-behavioral techniques, such as cognitive restructuring, to challenge negative sleep thoughts. Establish a calming pre-sleep routine, reduce screen time in the evening, and practice relaxation exercises.

- **Stay Asleep All Night** – Create a sleep-conducive environment using white noise machines, adjust room temperature for comfort, and align your sleep schedule with natural 90-minute sleep cycles to minimize nighttime awakenings.
- **Handle Nighttime Awakenings** – Stay calm if you wake up. Avoid checking the clock to reduce anxiety and use deep breathing or visualization techniques to help you drift back to sleep.
- **Manage Nightmares** – Use imagery rehearsal therapy to rewrite recurring nightmares, practice stress-reducing activities like meditation, and avoid heavy meals, caffeine, and alcohol before bedtime.
- **Naturally Address Sleep Apnea** – Lose weight if needed, sleep on your side to keep airways open, use positional therapy devices, and incorporate breathing exercises. Seek medical advice if symptoms persist for potential CPAP therapy.
- **Improve Sleep with Sexual Activity** – Engage in sexual activity (alone or with a partner) to promote relaxation through the release of hormones like oxytocin, prolactin, and endorphins, all of which reduce stress and enhance sleep quality.
- **Sleep Better While Traveling** – Choose window seats, wear comfortable layers, and use travel accessories like neck pillows and noise-canceling headphones. Manage jet lag by adjusting your sleep schedule before travel and seeking natural light upon arrival.
- **Cope with Sleep Paralysis** – Maintain a consistent sleep routine, use cognitive-behavioral therapy to reduce anxiety, and practice mindfulness techniques to stay calm during episodes. Consult a specialist if episodes become frequent or distressing.

6

NUTRITION AND SLEEP SYNERGY

> *"What you eat doesn't just fuel your day—it shapes your night. Balanced nutrition is key to restorative sleep."*
>
> — DR. MICHAEL BREUS

I magine a night where sleep comes easily, and the morning finds you refreshed and ready to seize the day. The key to such restful nights is often in your bedtime routine and the nutrients you consume throughout the day. Just as a car requires the right fuel to run smoothly, your body needs specific vitamins and minerals to support the complex sleep processes. Each nutrient is vital in ensuring your body can relax and rejuvenate at night, building a foundation for energy and productivity when you wake.

SLEEP-SUPPORTIVE NUTRIENTS

Magnesium stands out as a powerful ally in the quest for restful sleep. It is known for relaxing muscles and calming the nervous system. This essential mineral helps regulate neurotransmitters, the chemicals that transmit messages between your brain and body, reducing stress and promoting relaxation. When magnesium levels are sufficient, your body can more easily transition into restfulness, reducing the likelihood of nighttime awakenings. Add leafy greens like spinach and kale to incorporate magnesium into your diet. These greens are rich in magnesium and offer many other health benefits, making them a smart choice for any meal. Seeds and nuts, such as almonds and pumpkin seeds, are also excellent sources of magnesium and can be enjoyed as snacks or sprinkled over salads for added crunch and nutrition.

Vitamin B6 plays a crucial role in melatonin production, the hormone responsible for regulating sleep-wake cycles. Without adequate B6, your body may struggle to produce enough melatonin, leading to sleep onset and maintenance difficulties. Foods rich in vitamin B6 include whole grains, meats, vegetables, and fruits. By ensuring a varied and balanced diet, you can support your body's natural ability to produce melatonin and settle into sleep more easily. Consider incorporating whole grain cereals for breakfast, enjoying a piece of fruit as an afternoon snack, or adding vegetables like bell peppers and carrots to your dinner plate. This approach boosts your B6 intake and enhances overall dietary quality.

Calcium is another essential nutrient that supports sleep and is known for regulating sleep cycles. It aids in the production of melatonin and other neurotransmitters that facilitate sleep. Dairy products such as milk, yogurt, and cheese are well-known sources of calcium. Including these foods in your daily meals can ensure that your body has the calcium it needs to promote restful sleep. If dairy isn't part of your diet, consider alternatives like fortified plant-based milk or leafy greens such as broccoli and bok choy, which also provide calcium.

Omega-3 fatty acids, often found in fish oil supplements, are vital for maintaining healthy sleep patterns. These fats contribute to the regulation of neurotransmitters and reduce inflammation, which can interfere with sleep if left unchecked. Incorporating omega-3-rich foods like salmon, mackerel, or flaxseeds into your diet supports your body's ability to maintain a balanced sleep cycle. Regular consumption of omega-3s has been linked to improved sleep quality and duration, making them a worthy addition to your nutritional regimen.

Antioxidants play a critical role in sleep by reducing oxidative stress, which can disrupt sleep and lead to various health issues. Berries and nuts are rich in antioxidants and can be easily integrated into your diet. Enjoy a handful of berries as a sweet treat, or add them to your morning yogurt for a nutritious start to the day. Nuts, such as walnuts and pecans, offer a quick and satisfying snack that supports nighttime rest. These foods provide antioxidants and enhance overall health, making them a valuable component of a sleep-supportive diet.

Sleep-Supportive Foods Checklist

Consider incorporating these foods into your meals to boost sleep quality:

- **Leafy greens for magnesium:** Spinach, kale
- **Vitamin B6 sources:** Whole grains, meats, vegetables, fruits
- **Calcium-rich foods:** Dairy products, fortified plant-based milks, broccoli
- **Omega-3 sources:** Salmon, mackerel, flaxseeds
- **Antioxidant-rich foods:** Berries, nuts

You can also buy quality vitamin and mineral supplements from your local retailer. Personally, I've been taking various supplements for years, including each of the ones I've just listed.

By thoughtfully selecting and incorporating these nutrients into your daily diet, you lay the groundwork for achieving restorative sleep. The synergy between nutrition and sleep is immeasurable. You can enhance your nighttime rest and daytime vitality with the right nutritious choices.

TIMING YOUR MEALS FOR BETTER SLEEP

In the hustle and bustle of modern life, meal timing often gets overlooked, yet it plays a crucial role in how well you sleep. When you eat can be just as important as what you eat, especially when it comes to winding down for the night. Big, hearty dinners might seem satisfying, but consuming large meals close to bedtime can wreak havoc on your sleep cycles. Your digestive system ramps up to process the food, keeping your body awake when it should be powering down. This can lead to discomfort and restlessness, making it harder to fall asleep and stay asleep.

To optimize your sleep, consider adopting a consistent meal schedule. Eating at regular intervals helps regulate your body's internal clock, promoting a natural rhythm that aligns with your sleep-wake cycle. Aim to finish your last substantial meal at least two to three hours before bedtime. This gives your body ample time to digest, reducing the likelihood of sleep disturbances. If you are hungry in the evening, opt for light snacks that are easy to digest, such as those that can stave off hunger without overloading your system.

Intermittent fasting, particularly the 16/8 model, has been gaining attention for its potential benefits on sleep. This approach involves eating all your meals within eight hours, allowing your body to fast for the remaining 16 hours. The fasting period can help reset your circadian rhythms, aligning your body's internal clock with natural light and dark cycles. This synchronization can enhance sleep quality by promoting a more regular sleep pattern.

Research published in *Cell Metabolism* (2012) by Dr. Satchin Panda at the Salk Institute found that time-restricted eating, such as the 16/8 method, helps regulate the body's internal clock, leading to better digestion, stable energy levels, and improved sleep quality. Fasting for 16 hours allows the body to enter a state of ketosis, which burns stored fat for energy, promoting weight loss and better metabolic function.

A 2016 study in the *Journal of Obesity* found that participants practicing intermittent fasting experienced reduced nighttime hunger and more stable glucose levels, preventing energy crashes that can disrupt sleep. Additionally, research in *The Journal of Translational Medicine* (2019) showed that fasting reduces inflammation and lowers cortisol levels, decreasing stress and improving overall sleep quality.

By aligning eating patterns with the body's circadian rhythm, the 16/8 fasting method supports better digestion, hormonal balance, and deeper sleep, making it an effective tool for health and sleep optimization. However, it's important to approach fasting carefully and ensure that your dietary plan includes balanced, nutritious meals to support overall health.

If you're prone to late-night snacking, it's time to rethink your habits. Eating late at night can spike your blood sugar and insulin levels, making it difficult for your body to settle into a restful state.

By aligning your eating habits with your body's natural rhythms and nutrition needs, you create a supportive foundation for restful nights and productive days. The connection between what you eat, when you eat, and how you sleep is intense and underscores the importance of thoughtful meal preparations in your quest for better rest.

HERBAL REMEDIES FOR RESTFUL NIGHTS

For centuries, people have turned to natural remedies to support restful sleep, and today, herbal supplements offer a gentle, effective alternative to pharmaceuticals. Valerian root, widely celebrated for its relaxation and calming properties, is often the first defense against insomnia. This ancient herb works by increasing levels of gamma-aminobutyric acid (GABA) in the brain, a neurotransmitter that reduces nerve activity, promoting relaxation and ease. Unlike traditional sleep aids, valerian is non-addictive, making it a popular choice for those seeking natural solutions. Chamomile tea, another favorite remedy, is renowned for its mild sedative effects. Sipping warm chamomile tea before bed can become a soothing evening ritual.

The appeal of herbal remedies lies in their ability to promote sleep without the side effects often associated with prescription sleep aids, which can lead to dependency or grogginess the next day and leave you feeling worse rather than rested. Herbal options also tend to be gentler on the system. They work with your body's natural processes rather than overriding them. This makes herbs like valerian and chamomile excellent choices for those looking to improve sleep quality without the risk of addiction. While scientific studies on herbal efficacy can vary, many people find these natural treatments effective and comforting parts of their nightly routine.

Incorporating herbs into your bedtime routine can be a simple yet transformative practice. Instead of a tablet or capsule form, try herbal teas with chamomile and/or valerian about an hour before bed, which allows your body to better absorb their calming compounds.

If you prefer not to drink tea, consider using essential oils in your evening routine. We had discussed using essential oils in Chapter 2, and it's important to bring them up here in our full discussion on herbal remedies for sleep. As you may remember, I had mentioned that Lavender oil, known for its anxiety-reducing properties, can be diffused in the bedroom or applied to your pillowcase to create a calming environment. Similarly, passion-flower, often used to address sleep latency, can be taken as a supplement or tincture. This herb is also known for its ability to increase levels of GABA, helping reduce the time it takes to fall asleep.

Including herbs in your sleep strategy offers a natural, holistic approach to rest. Whether you choose to sip a warm cup of tea, breathe in the calming scent of essential oils, or take a supplement, these remedies can help create an environment where sleep comes naturally and peacefully.

MANAGING CAFFEINE AND SUGAR INTAKE

I've already discussed caffeine, but let's also review it here for your ease of reference. Sugar is often consumed with caffeine, so we can take a closer look at how they work to affect sleep in this section.

Caffeine, of course, is the quintessential pick-me-up, a staple in countless morning routines. Yet, its impact on sleep is often disruptive. As a central nervous system stimulant, caffeine increases alertness, making it difficult for your body to wind down at night. This is mainly due to its half-life, which is the time it takes for half of the substance to be eliminated from your system. Caffeine's half-life can range from three to seven hours, meaning that a late afternoon cup of coffee could still affect your body when it's time to hit the hay. This lingering presence can extend sleep latency, the time it takes to fall asleep, causing a restless night. Over time, this sleep disruption can accumulate, leaving you exhausted during the day and reaching for even more caffeine to compensate.

Reducing caffeine intake can significantly improve your sleep quality, and there are practical steps you can take to cut back without sacrificing your morning ritual. One effective strategy is to switch to decaffeinated options gradually. Start by mixing regular and decaf coffee, slowly increasing the proportion of decaf until you've weaned yourself off the caffeine buzz. Alternatively, explore other caffeine-free beverages, such as herbal teas, that offer comforting warmth without the stimulant effects. It's also wise to establish a caffeine curfew, cutting off consumption after midday to give your body ample time to metabolize the caffeine before bedtime. This simple shift can make a noticeable difference in how easily you fall asleep and how rested you feel the next day.

Sugar, much like Caffeine, can play havoc with sleep. Consuming sugary foods or drinks may lead to a quick energy boost, but they also cause blood sugar levels to spike and crash. This rollercoaster effect can disrupt your sleep, causing you to wake up in the middle of the night or experience restless sleep. The body works hard to regulate these fluctuations, which can interfere with the natural processes that promote deep, restorative rest. For those who find themselves reaching for sweets out of habit or stress, understanding the impact of sugar on sleep can be a compelling reason to rethink those late-night cravings.

To satisfy a sweet tooth without compromising sleep, consider healthier alternatives that won't send your blood sugar levels on a wild ride. Natural sweeteners like honey can offer a gentle, more stable energy release compared to refined sugars. A small spoonful of honey in a cup of warm milk or herbal tea provides the perfect balance of sweetness and comfort. Fruit-based desserts are another excellent option, combining natural sugars with fiber and nutrients. A baked apple with a sprinkle of cinnamon or a bowl of fresh berries can be satisfying and nourishing without the sleep-disrupting consequences of processed sweets.

Navigating the intricate relationship between diet and sleep involves recognizing caffeine and sugar's roles in your nightly rest. By moderating these substances and making thoughtful dietary choices, you create an environment that supports better sleep. Small changes in what you consume and when can significantly improve how you feel at night and throughout the day.

HYDRATION AND SLEEP

The relationship between hydration and sleep is often overlooked, yet it plays a critical role in maintaining continuous, restful sleep. Water is essential for every cell in your body, and being well-hydrated helps ensure optimal functioning of your body's systems, including those that regulate sleep. Proper hydration aids in maintaining a stable internal environment, which is crucial for the body's natural sleep cycles. When your body lacks sufficient water, it can lead to dehydration, causing discomfort, headaches, or dry mouth, all of which can disrupt your sleep. Furthermore, hydration affects the balance of electrolytes—minerals like sodium, potassium, and calcium—essential for conducting electrical impulses in your body. These electrolytes help maintain the body's fluid balance, nerve function, and muscle contractions, all vital for sound sleep.

Coconut water is an excellent natural source of electrolytes, particularly potassium, which can aid in maintaining hydration and supporting muscle relaxation. Sipping coconut water during the day can be a refreshing way to replenish electrolytes, especially after physical activity or on hot days. By ensuring that your body has the right balance of electrolytes, you create a stable internal environment that supports restful sleep.

Establishing a hydration schedule throughout the day can help you achieve and maintain optimal hydration levels, minimizing the risk of waking up parched in the middle of the night. Start your day with a glass of water to kick-start your body's hydration, and then continue to drink small amounts regularly throughout the day. Consuming water at intervals can ensure that your body remains hydrated without overwhelming your system with large volumes at once. Hydrating foods, such as fruits and vegetables, can also contribute to your daily water intake, providing hydration and essential nutrients.

Balancing hydration and avoiding frequent nighttime bathroom trips requires a thoughtful approach to fluid intake. While it's essential to stay hydrated, drinking large amounts of fluid too close to bedtime can interrupt your sleep as your body prompts you to visit the bathroom. To strike the right balance, consider limiting your fluid intake at least an hour before you plan to sleep. Then, focus on hydrating well during the earlier parts of the day, allowing your body to benefit from the fluids without compromising your sleep quality.

Paying attention to your body's hydration needs and managing your fluid and electrolyte balance can enhance your sleep quality and overall well-being. Minor adjustments in how and when you hydrate can lead to more consistent, uninterrupted sleep, allowing you to wake up refreshed and ready to take on the day.

FOOD SENSITIVITIES AND SLEEP DISRUPTIONS

Sleep, a fundamental pillar of health, can be disrupted by what you eat, particularly if you're sensitive to certain foods. Though often overlooked, food sensitivities can play a significant role in sleep disturbances. Common culprits include gluten and dairy, triggering inflammatory responses in susceptible individuals. The discomfort from such reactions might not always be immediate. Still, it can manifest later, affecting your ability to fall or stay asleep. If you find yourself tossing and turning at night, it might be worth examining your diet for potential sensitivities. Gluten in wheat, barley, and rye can lead to digestive discomfort, while dairy might cause bloating or congestion. These physical discomforts can interrupt the deep, restful sleep your body craves.

I often take digestive enzymes when I eat certain heavier foods, which can help with that bloated or heavy feeling in my stomach. Like the other supplements I mentioned, quality enzymes can be purchased at your local retailer. Talk with the in-store expert for advice on which brand will do the best job for you.

Identifying and managing dietary sensitivities requires a bit of detective work. One effective strategy is an elimination diet in which you remove potential triggers from your meals for a period and then gradually reintroduce them. This method allows you to observe any changes in your sleep patterns or overall well-being, helping you pinpoint the foods that might be causing issues. Keeping a food and sleep journal can further aid this process. By tracking what you eat and noting your sleep quality each night, you can start to spot patterns and correlations. This documentation can be invaluable in identifying hidden sensitivities that might otherwise go unnoticed.

Histamine, a compound found in various foods, can also impact sleep quality. In some individuals, consuming histamine-rich foods can lead to increased wakefulness or disrupted sleep. Aged cheeses, fermented products like sauerkraut, and certain cured meats are known for high histamine levels. These foods can trigger allergic-like reactions or exacerbate existing sensitivities, creating a state of heightened alertness when you should be winding down. If you suspect histamine might be affecting your sleep, consider reducing or avoiding these foods, especially before bedtime.

Fortunately, there are alternative foods that can help you circumvent these sensitivities without sacrificing variety or flavor. Plant-based milks such as almond, soy, or oat milk can serve as excellent substitutes for those with dairy sensitivities. These options provide a creamy texture and are fortified with essential nutrients like calcium and vitamin D, supporting overall health. Exploring gluten-free grains like quinoa, rice, and buckwheat can offer delicious and nutritious alternatives for gluten-sensitive individuals. These versatile grains can be incorporated into various dishes, from hearty breakfasts to wholesome dinners.

Addressing food sensitivities is about more than just avoiding discomfort; it's about optimizing your sleep environment from the inside out. By being mindful of what you consume and how it affects your body, you set the stage for better rest and rejuvenation. As you navigate these dietary changes, remember that minor adjustments can significantly improve how you feel at night and throughout the day. By aligning your diet with your body's unique needs, you enhance your sleep quality and contribute to a healthier, more balanced lifestyle.

As you reflect on the foods you consume and their impact on your sleep, consider how these choices integrate into your broader wellness plan. Nutrition is just one piece of the puzzle, a pivotal component that complements other lifestyle factors in your pursuit of restorative rest.

Summary:

- **Prioritize Sleep-Supportive Nutrients** – Incorporate magnesium (leafy greens, nuts), vitamin B6 (whole grains, vegetables), calcium (dairy, fortified plant-based milk), omega-3s (salmon, flaxseeds), and antioxidants (berries, nuts) to support melatonin production and relaxation.
- **Optimize Meal Timing for Sleep** – Avoid large meals within 2–3 hours before bedtime to prevent digestion-related sleep disruptions. Consider intermittent fasting (for example, the 16/8 method) to regulate circadian rhythms and improve your sleep quality.
- **Use Herbal Remedies for Natural Relaxation** – To enhance relaxation without dependency, drink chamomile or valerian tea before bed, diffuse lavender essential oil, or take passionflower supplements.
- **Manage Caffeine and Sugar Intake** – Cut off caffeine by early afternoon and reduce sugar consumption to prevent energy crashes that disrupt sleep. Switch to herbal teas, honey, or fruit-based desserts for better sleep stability.
- **Stay Hydrated Without Nighttime Disruptions** – Drink water throughout the day but limit fluid intake an hour before bed to avoid frequent awakenings. Maintain electrolyte balance with coconut water or hydrating fruits.
- **Identify and Avoid Food Sensitivities** – Watch for gluten, dairy, and histamine-rich foods that may cause

inflammation or sleeplessness. Keep a food and sleep journal to track potential dietary triggers.

- **Choose Smart Food Alternatives** – Replace dairy with plant-based milk, gluten with quinoa or rice, and processed sweets with natural options like nuts and fruits to maintain a balanced diet while supporting restful sleep.

7

SLEEP SOLUTIONS FOR FAMILIES

"Good sleep habits start at home. When parents model healthy sleep routines, children are more likely to follow."

— DR. JODI MINDELL (SLEEP RESEARCHER)

I magine the familiar scene of trying to get everyone in your household to wind down for the night. The kids are still buzzing with energy, and you find yourself juggling between calming them down and preparing for another busy day ahead. In such a whirlwind, establishing a family sleep routine may seem daunting. Yet, such an effort holds the key to transforming chaotic evenings into peaceful ones where everyone benefits from restful sleep. A unified family sleep schedule ensures that everyone gets the sleep they need and creates an environment in which predictability and reduced stress reign supreme. When each family member knows what to expect as bedtime approaches, a sense of security and calm prevails, making the transition from day to night smoother for all.

Setting a collective bedtime for children is foundational to this routine. Children thrive on consistency, and a regular bedtime helps regulate their internal clocks, making it easier for them to fall asleep and wake up refreshed. Consider aligning adult schedules with the children's routines as much as possible. This helps reinforce the importance of sleep for everyone in the household and models healthy sleep habits for your kids. When children see adults prioritizing sleep, it underscores its value and encourages them to follow suit. Synchronizing these schedules can also carve out more family time, allowing everyone to connect and unwind, a critical component of a healthy family dynamic.

Planning nightly activities that promote winding down can further enhance the effectiveness of your family sleep routine. Reading storybooks together can become a cherished ritual, offering a moment of calm and connection before bed. A well-told story can transport your family to a world of imagination while gently easing the transition to sleep. Beyond storytelling, engaging in family meditation sessions can be immensely beneficial. Simple guided breathing exercises or mindfulness practices can help everyone, regardless of age, to center themselves and release the day's tensions. These activities prepare the mind for rest and build a sense of togetherness, reinforcing the collective nature of the family routine.

Flexibility within the routine is essential to accommodate the diverse needs of each family member without disrupting the overall schedule. While consistency is critical, allowing for slight adjustments on weekends or special occasions can prevent the routine from becoming rigid or burdensome. Perhaps bedtime can be extended by half an hour on a Friday night for a family movie, or the schedule can be adapted for a special event. This adaptability ensures that the routine remains sustainable and respectful of individual needs, keeping everyone engaged and committed.

Communication and teamwork play pivotal roles in establishing a successful family sleep routine. Involve all family members in the planning process to foster buy-in and cooperation. Hold family meetings to discuss bedtime preferences, where everyone can shape the routine. This collaborative approach empowers children and adults, making each person more likely to adhere to the agreed-on schedule. Through open dialogue and shared decision-making, you create a supportive environment where everyone's sleep needs are valued and prioritized.

Family Sleep Routine Checklist

To guide your family in establishing a successful sleep routine, consider the following checklist:

- Set a consistent bedtime for children and align adult schedules with theirs.
- Incorporate calming activities like reading storybooks or family meditation sessions before bed.
- Maintain flexibility within the routine to accommodate individual needs and special occasions.
- Encourage open communication and involve all family members in establishing the routine.

By embracing these strategies, you can transform your family's evenings into a time of tranquility and connection, paving the way for restful nights and energized days.

INTRODUCING SLEEP RITUALS FOR CHILDREN

Creating bedtime rituals for children can be a magical way to transition them from the active play of their day to the calm needed for a good night's sleep. These rituals act as gentle cues, signaling young minds and bodies that it's time to wind down. Calming gentle lullabies or soft music, which can lull them to sleep with the power of melody, can be a powerful ally. Familiar notes and lyrics create an auditory environment of reassurance and peace, making the transition from wakefulness to slumber seamless and comforting.

Establishing these rituals doesn't have to be complex. Start with a warm bath, which helps relax their muscles and signals the start of the bedtime process. Follow this with quiet activities encouraging relaxation, such as drawing or puzzles, which can help them wind down further. It's crucial to set a specific order to bedtime tasks, creating a predictable pattern that their bodies will soon associate with sleep. This might look like a sequence of brushing teeth, putting on pajamas, and settling into bed with a favorite stuffed animal. This structured approach reinforces the family's routine, making it easier for children to follow and anticipate what comes next while teaching them the value of planning and responsibility.

Each child is unique, so tailoring these bedtime rituals to their age and developmental stage is essential. Incorporating some imaginary play can be a delightful way to ease into bedtime for toddlers. A plush toy could become a bedtime buddy, joining them as they embark on a calming adventure under the covers. This playful element speaks to their imagination, transforming bedtime into a positive experience rather than a chore. As children grow older, their needs change, and so should their rituals. Guided relaxation exercises can be introduced to older children, teaching them to focus on their breath or visualize a peaceful setting. These exercises can help them learn how to manage stress and anxiety while fostering a sense of calm and control over their bedtime routine.

Involving children in creating their bedtime rituals can significantly enhance their effectiveness. Let them choose the storybook for the evening or decide the order of their bedtime activities. This involvement encourages them to take responsibility for their own sleep hygiene, reinforcing the importance of routine. Additionally, they should be involved in setting up their sleep environment. Let them arrange their pillows and blankets or choose a nightlight. This participation makes bedtime more engaging, fosters independence, and increases confidence in their ability to contribute to their own well-being.

MANAGING TEEN SLEEP CHALLENGES

Teenagers live in a world of constant growth and change, and their sleep needs are no exception. As they navigate these transformative years, their biological changes significantly impact their sleep patterns. Many teens experience a shift in their internal body clocks, known as delayed sleep phase syndrome, which causes them to naturally feel awake later at night and sleepy later in the morning. This shift often conflicts with early school start times, making it difficult for teens to get the rest they need. During adolescence, growth and development increase the need for sleep, with experts recommending 8–10 hours per night. However, school demands, social activities, and the lure of screens often eat into these precious hours, leaving many teens chronically sleep-deprived.

Encouraging healthy sleep habits in teenagers can be challenging but not impossible. To help your teen balance their daily activities with adequate rest, start by setting a consistent sleep schedule. Consistency is key in regulating their internal clock, so encourage them to go to bed and wake up simultaneously every day, even on weekends. Educate them about the effects of screen time on sleep, highlighting how the blue light from devices can interfere with melatonin production. Encourage them to power down screens at least an hour before bedtime, using this time for relaxing activities like reading or listening to music. By helping them understand the impact of their choices, you empower them to prioritize their sleep health.

School and social pressures can weigh heavily on a teen's sleep, adding layers of stress that disrupt their ability to rest. The pressure to excel academically can lead to late-night study sessions. At the same time, the desire to stay connected with friends can result in endless scrolling through social media. Both can erode valuable sleep time. Instead, teens can be encouraged to practice stress management techniques such as mindfulness or engaging in physical activities they enjoy, as exercise can be a powerful stress reliever. Such guidance helps them develop time management skills to balance homework and leisure activities more effectively.

Open communication about sleep with your teenager is crucial. Create a supportive environment where they feel comfortable discussing their sleep habits and needs. Ask open-ended questions about how they feel in the mornings or if they've noticed any patterns in their sleep. This dialogue can provide insights into their challenges, allowing you to work together on solutions. Encourage collaborative problem-solving, where you brainstorm on strategies to improve their sleep. Whether adjusting their evening routine or finding better ways to manage stress, involving them fosters a sense of agency and responsibility. This shared approach helps them develop healthier sleep habits and strengthens your relationship through mutual understanding and respect.

SLEEP SUPPORT FOR NEW PARENTS

Welcoming a new baby into the world brings joy and love. The increasingly busy days to follow also usher in a period of profound sleep disruption for parents. The demands of infant care, from midnight feedings to soothing a fussy baby, often leave new parents deprived of sleep. This lack of rest can take a toll both physically and emotionally. Sleep deprivation affects mood, making you more irritable and prone to mood swings. It can also impair cognitive function, leading to forgetfulness and difficulty concentrating during the day. The constant cycle of sleep interruption leaves you exhausted and challenged to find the energy needed for fully enjoying the early days of parenthood.

To combat fragmented sleep effects, optimizing rest whenever possible is crucial. One practical strategy is to sleep when the baby sleeps. It might sound simple, but grabbing those precious moments of rest during your baby's naps can result in significant recovery over time. Additionally, sharing nighttime responsibilities with a partner can alleviate the burden. Divide tasks such as feedings and diaper changes so each parent can rest at night. For breastfeeding mothers, consider pumping milk in advance, allowing your partner to handle some feedings and give you a chance to sleep uninterrupted.

Support systems are invaluable for new parents navigating sleep deprivation. Family, friends, and community resources can provide much-needed relief. Don't hesitate to seek help from family members or hire childcare services for a few hours to rest. Many communities offer support groups where parents can share experiences and advice, which fosters a network of understanding and assistance. Leveraging these resources can give you the necessary breaks to recharge, allowing you to face parenting challenges with renewed energy and patience.

Managing stress and fatigue is also crucial for new parents. Incorporating relaxation methods into your routine can significantly reduce stress levels and improve overall energy. Mindfulness exercises I've discussed, such as deep breathing or short meditation sessions, can help center your mind and alleviate the mental strain of parenting. These practices encourage you to focus on the present moment, reducing anxiety and promoting a sense of calm. Short, restorative naps during the day can also make a world of difference. Even a brief 20-minute nap can refresh your mind and body, improving alertness and mood. Prioritize these moments of rest whenever possible, recognizing that self-care is essential for your well-being and your ability to care for your baby effectively.

ENCOURAGING INDEPENDENT SLEEP IN CHILDREN

Imagine the satisfaction of watching your child drift off to sleep, their breathing steady and calm, without needing you by their side. Encouraging independent sleep in children is about more than just getting a good night's rest for yourself. It builds their confidence and fosters self-reliance, essential traits that will serve them well throughout life. Children who learn to fall asleep on their own are less likely to wake up during the night, searching for reassurance. This autonomy leads to more restful nights and helps them develop a sense of achievement and security in their ability to manage bedtime independently.

The transition to independent sleep doesn't have to be abrupt or challenging. Start by gradually reducing your presence at bedtime. If you usually stay at bedside until your child falls asleep, try sitting in a chair by the door instead. Over time, move the chair further away, eventually saying goodnight at the door. This gentle withdrawal helps them adjust without feeling abandoned. Comfort objects can also be invaluable during this transition. A cherished stuffed animal or a favorite blanket can provide their needed security. These items are tangible reminders of your presence, offering comfort and reassurance throughout the night.

Positive reinforcement plays a significant role in promoting sleep independence. Children thrive on encouragement and praise, so consider using a reward system to celebrate their successes. Sticker charts are a simple yet effective tool. Each night your child goes to bed without needing you to stay can earn them a sticker, leading to a small reward after collecting a set number of them. This system makes the process fun and engaging; celebrate their progress enthusiastically, reinforcing their efforts and boosting their confidence in their ability to sleep independently.

Of course, the path to independent sleep isn't always smooth, and you may encounter setbacks. Nighttime fears are common hurdles, such as fear of the dark or monsters under the bed. Address these concerns with empathy and understanding. Reassure your child that they are safe and explore creative solutions to alleviate their fears, such as using a nightlight or engaging in a "monster hunt" to show them there's nothing to fear.

Consistency in routines is key. Stick to the established bedtime routine as closely as possible, even when challenges arise. This consistency provides structure and predictability, helping them feel secure while reinforcing the routine as a natural part of their day.

Encouraging independent sleep in children is a journey filled with small victories and learning moments. By fostering confidence and self-reliance, you empower your children to embrace bedtime with courage, preparing them for many restful nights and bright mornings ahead.

HANDLING BEDTIME RESISTANCE

Bedtime resistance in children is a challenge many parents face, often leaving them feeling frustrated and helpless as sleep time approaches. Children might resist going to bed for several reasons and understanding them can be key to resolving the issue. One common factor is the "fear of missing out." Children, curious by nature, often believe that the world continues to buzz with excitement and adventure even as they lie in bed. This belief can lead to reluctance to settle down, as they feel they might miss something important or fun.

Additionally, anxiety or fear of the dark can play a significant role. Shadows turn into imaginary creatures, and unfamiliar sounds become threats in the stillness of the night, making children anxious about being alone in their rooms. These fears can create a strong resistance to bedtime as the comfort of daylight fades.

Setting clear and consistent expectations is crucial to address and reduce bedtime resistance. Children thrive on routine and understanding what is expected of them. Communicate the importance of bedtime and the benefits of a good night's sleep, explaining how it helps them grow and prepare for the next day's fun. Additionally, activities such as taking a warm bath, dimming the lights, or playing soft music can help children wind down.

Patience and empathy are vital when dealing with bedtime resistance. Listening to your child's concerns and fears with an open heart is important. Empathetic listening involves validating their feelings and acknowledging that their worries or reluctance are real and significant to them. Offering comfort and reassurance can go a long way in easing their anxieties. For instance, you might stay with them for a few extra minutes, talking about their day or sharing a reassuring story. This helps them feel understood and strengthens your shared bond, creating a sense of security and trust.

Creativity can be your ally in making bedtime an appealing and enjoyable experience. Introducing themed story nights can turn

SLEEP SOLUTIONS FOR FAMILIES | 121

bedtime into an anticipated adventure. Each night could bring a new theme—be it pirates, outer space, or enchanted forests— with stories and discussions revolving around these topics. Bedtime games that promote relaxation can also be effective. Simple games like "I Spy" with calming elements or "Count the Stars" can help shift their focus from reluctance to relaxation. These fun, engaging activities provide a gentle bridge from the day's excitement to the tranquility of sleep, transforming bedtime from a battleground into a cherished part of their daily routine.

Summary:

- **Establish a Unified Family Sleep Routine** – Set consistent bedtimes for children and align adult schedules to model healthy sleep habits. Incorporate calming activities like storytelling or family meditation to create a peaceful transition from day to night.
- **Create Engaging Sleep Rituals for Children** – Introduce predictable bedtime routines like warm baths, quiet play, and lullabies. Tailor rituals based on age, incorporating guided relaxation for older kids and imaginative play for toddlers to foster calm.
- **Manage Teen Sleep Challenges** – Acknowledge teens' natural shift toward later bedtimes due to biological changes. Encourage consistent sleep schedules, limit screen time before bed, and introduce stress management techniques to balance academic and social demands.
- **Support New Parents Through Sleep Deprivation** – Share nighttime duties, sleep when the baby sleeps, and seek help from family or support groups. Short restorative naps and mindfulness practices can combat fatigue and maintain energy levels.

- **Encourage Independent Sleep in Children** – Gradually reduce bedtime presence and use comfort objects like stuffed animals. Introduce reward systems (e.g., sticker charts) to reinforce sleep independence while addressing nighttime fears with empathy.
- **Handle Bedtime Resistance with Creativity** – Reduce your children's "fear of missing out" and anxious feelings about darkness by maintaining a calm bedtime routine and validating their concerns. Make bedtime fun with themed story nights or relaxation-focused games like "Count the Stars."
- **Foster Communication and Flexibility** – Hold family meetings to discuss sleep routines, fostering buy-in from all members. Maintain routine consistency while allowing for occasional flexibility on weekends or special occasions.

8

LONG-TERM SLEEP OPTIMIZATION

"Sleep isn't a luxury; it's a long-term investment in your health, performance, and well-being."

— DR. MATTHEW WALKER

The secret to this refreshed state lies in what you do at night and how you continuously improve your sleep quality over time. As we delve into the strategies for long-term sleep optimization, we explore how technology can be a powerful ally in your quest for better rest. Sleep tracking has become a valuable tool for those striving to understand and enhance their slumber. By capturing a snapshot of your nightly rhythms, modern methods offer insights that were once the domain of specialized sleep labs.

The world of sleep tracking is vast, with a variety of devices and apps designed to monitor your sleep patterns. Wearable sleep trackers, often in the form of smartwatches or fitness bands, provide a convenient way to track your sleep. These gadgets measure heart rate, movement, and even temperature, offering a comprehensive view of your sleep cycles. They are particularly useful for tracking how long you stay in each sleep stage and how often you wake up at night. Smartphone applications are another option, transforming your phone into a sleep-monitoring tool. These apps utilize your phone's sensors to detect movement and sound, capturing data that helps paint a picture of your sleep quality.

Selecting the right sleep-tracking tool involves considering your personal needs and preferences. Look for features that align with your goals, such as heart rate monitoring, which can provide insights into how restful your sleep is, or sleep stage analysis, which breaks down the time you spend in light, deep, and REM sleep. User-friendly interfaces and detailed reports can make interpreting your data easier and track progress over time.

When using apps and devices, you will want to review their privacy policies and data security that are in place to protect your sensitive information. There are several useful sleep tracking and assistance options in this realm, which makes looking into them worth your time. For example, I personally use an Oura Ring and like it a lot, while my wife uses a Google watch.

Interpreting the data collected by these devices is key to making meaningful changes. Start by recognizing patterns of sleep disruption. Are you waking up frequently during the night? Is your sleep fragmented or cut short? Understanding these patterns can help you identify the underlying causes of poor sleep, such as stress, diet, or environmental factors. Correlating sleep data with lifestyle changes can provide further insights. For instance, if you notice improved sleep after reducing caffeine intake or adopting a relaxing bedtime routine, you can use this information to reinforce positive habits.

Regularly reviewing and adjusting your sleep strategies based on your collected data is crucial for continuous improvement. Monthly sleep audits allow you to assess your progress and make necessary adjustments. Consider setting realistic goals based on your tracked data, such as aiming for a consistent bedtime or reducing the number of nighttime awakenings. By approaching sleep optimization as an ongoing process, you empower yourself to make informed decisions that enhance your sleep quality over time.

Sleep Tracking Journal

Start a sleep-tracking journal alongside your digital tools. Record your nightly data, noting any lifestyle changes or events that might have influenced your sleep. Reflect on patterns and set monthly goals to foster continuous improvement. Use this book as a personal guide to refine your sleep habits and celebrate your progress toward deeper, more restorative sleep.

VIRTUAL SLEEP COACHES

While traditional sleep therapy can be effective, it's often expensive, time-consuming, or difficult to access. This is where virtual sleep coaches come in—digital tools designed to guide users through personalized sleep improvement programs using science-backed techniques. These platforms combine technology with behavioral science to help individuals optimize their sleep patterns, and studies show they can be highly effective.

Virtual sleep coaches typically use a combination of data tracking, personalized feedback, and behavioral interventions to improve sleep habits. These programs often start by assessing a user's current sleep patterns, usually through sleep diaries, questionnaires, or integrations with wearable devices like Fitbit or Apple Watch. Based on this data, the coach identifies problematic behaviors—such as inconsistent sleep schedules, excessive screen time, or caffeine consumption—and provides customized recommendations.

Many virtual sleep coaches are built around cognitive behavioral therapy for insomnia (CBT-I), the gold standard treatment for chronic sleep issues. A meta-analysis published in the *Annals of Internal Medicine* (2015) found that CBT-I is more effective than sleep medications in improving sleep quality and has longer-lasting results. Virtual sleep coaches make CBT-I techniques more accessible by delivering them digitally, often through interactive modules, guided exercises, and regular check-ins.

Popular Virtual Sleep Coach Apps and Platforms

- **Sleepio:** Sleepio is one of the most well-known digital sleep coaching platforms developed by sleep scientists. It offers a six-week CBT-I program that uses an AI-driven virtual coach to guide users through techniques like stimulus control, sleep restriction, and relaxation exercises. A study published in *JAMA Psychiatry* (2016) showed that 76% of Sleepio users experienced significant improvements in sleep quality, demonstrating its effectiveness as a digital intervention.
- **BetterSleep (formerly Relax Melodies):** While BetterSleep offers a variety of relaxing soundscapes and meditations, it also includes personalized sleep programs. The app uses your sleep goals and habits to suggest tailored bedtime routines, mindfulness exercises, and breathing techniques to promote better sleep.

- **Somryst:** This prescription digital therapeutic is FDA-approved and delivers CBT-I for people with chronic insomnia. It offers structured programs and progress tracking, allowing users to monitor their improvements over time. Studies have shown Somryst to effectively reduce the time it takes to fall asleep and improve overall sleep duration.
- **Pzizz:** This app uses a mix of binaural beats, guided imagery, and soundscapes to help users fall asleep faster and stay asleep longer. It also adjusts its recommendations based on user feedback and sleep patterns.

The success of virtual sleep coaches is grounded in behavioral science and sleep hygiene principles. They use CBT-I techniques like stimulus control (associating the bed only with sleep), sleep restriction (limiting time in bed to increase sleep efficiency), and cognitive restructuring (challenging negative thoughts about sleep). These methods have been widely studied and proven effective for treating insomnia and other sleep disorders.

Moreover, virtual sleep coaches provide real-time feedback and accountability, which is crucial for behavior change. A study in *The Journal of Medical Internet Research* (2020) found that digital health interventions, including virtual sleep coaches, effectively improved sleep quality and duration, particularly because they allowed users to track progress and receive personalized guidance.

Virtual sleep coaches can offer an accessible, cost-effective way to improve sleep health. As research continues to support the effectiveness of digital sleep interventions, virtual sleep coaches are becoming an increasingly valuable tool for anyone looking to achieve consistent, restorative sleep.

INTEGRATING SLEEP WITH OVERALL WELLNESS

Sleep is a cornerstone of health, intricately woven into the broader fabric of wellness. It interacts seamlessly with nutrition, exercise, and mental well-being, creating a network that influences our daily lives. Quality sleep supports your immune system by promoting the production of cytokines, proteins that help fight infections and inflammation. Without sufficient sleep, your body's defense mechanism weakens, leaving you more susceptible to illnesses.

In the context of holistic health, sleep doesn't operate in isolation. It's a vital component of the mind-body connection, where mental and physical health are intertwined. Synergistic interactions between sleep, diet, and exercise can create a positive feedback loop, where improvements in one area bolster the others. For example, better sleep increases your energy levels, making engaging in regular exercise more manageable, which can lead to even better sleep.

Balancing sleep with other wellness goals requires a thoughtful approach. Consider how you can coordinate your workout schedule with your sleep patterns. Morning exercise can boost your alertness for the day, while evening yoga can help you wind down. Pay attention to how your body responds to different types of exercise and adjust your routine accordingly. It's also essential to manage stress through relaxation techniques like meditation or deep breathing, which can promote restful sleep.

The benefits of improved sleep extend beyond just feeling refreshed. Increased energy levels with restorative rest make you more likely to engage in physical activities, which further supports cardiovascular health and weight management. Better sleep also sharpens your mental acuity, improving focus and productivity at work. Emotionally, it can lead to a more stable mood, reducing the risk of anxiety and depression. These improvements create a cycle of wellness, where each component supports and enhances the others, leading to a healthier, more fulfilling life.

Embracing sleep as a fundamental pillar of health is not just about getting enough rest. It's about recognizing its role in the broader context of wellness and making conscious choices that align with your overall health objectives.

THE ROLE OF EXERCISE IN SLEEP QUALITY

Physical activity has a profound influence on how well you sleep. When you exercise regularly, you enhance the structure and pattern of your sleep cycles. Notably, exercise helps increase the duration of deep sleep, the most restorative stage in which the body repairs itself and builds energy for the day ahead. As you work out, your body's temperature rises. As it cools down post-exercise, it signals to your brain that it's time to wind down, thus facilitating sleep onset. This cooling process can help you fall asleep quicker and stay asleep longer, resulting in a more restful night.

The intensity of your exercise routine also plays a role in sleep quality. Moderate exercise is generally beneficial for improving sleep patterns, as it helps reduce the time it takes to fall asleep and decreases the number of awakenings during the night. While it can enhance sleep quality by increasing the amount of slow-wave sleep, it may also raise your heart rate and adrenaline levels, making it harder to wind down if done too late in the evening. Find a balance that works for you and ensure that your exercise routine complements your sleep habits rather than disrupts them.

Consistency and variety in your exercise habits are key to reaping long-term benefits. Aim to engage in physical activity most days of the week, mixing aerobic exercises like running, swimming, or cycling with strength training and flexibility exercises. This variety keeps your workouts interesting and caters to different aspects of physical fitness, supporting overall health. Regular exercise encourages better sleep patterns, and quality sleep gives you the vitality needed to maintain an active lifestyle. Integrating diverse workouts into your routine builds a sustainable habit supporting your physical and sleep health.

Establishing an exercise routine that supports sleep requires listening to your body and understanding its rhythms. Pay attention to how different types of exercise affect your sleep and adjust accordingly. Whether you're a morning runner or an evening yogi, finding a routine that fits your lifestyle and enhances your sleep quality is key. Exercise is not just about physical fitness; it's a holistic practice that influences how you feel, function, and rest. By prioritizing physical activity, you lay the foundation for a healthier, more balanced life, where each workout brings you closer to achieving your sleep and wellness goals.

LOSE WEIGHT WHILE YOU SLEEP

It might sound too good to be true, but your body does more than rest while you sleep—it actively regulates hormones, repairs tissues, and even burns calories. Scientific research has shown that optimizing your sleep environment and habits can significantly influence your metabolism and fat-burning potential. From balancing hormones to adjusting room temperature, sleep plays a vital role in weight management.

One of the most critical links between sleep and weight loss is hormonal regulation; two key hormones, ghrelin and leptin, control hunger and satiety. Ghrelin signals hunger to the brain, while leptin tells you when you're full. When you don't get enough sleep, ghrelin levels rise, and leptin levels fall, leading to increased appetite and cravings, particularly for high-calorie, carb-heavy foods. A landmark study from the University of Chicago (2004) revealed that sleep-deprived individuals experienced a 24% increase in hunger, especially for sugary snacks.

Sleep deprivation also disrupts insulin sensitivity, which affects how efficiently your body processes glucose. Poor insulin sensitivity makes it easier for your body to store fat, particularly around the abdomen. Research published in *Annals of Internal Medicine* (2010) showed that just four nights of restricted sleep led to a 30% drop in insulin sensitivity, increasing the risk of weight gain and metabolic disorders.

Sleep quality plays a role in how efficiently your body burns calories. A study published in *Obesity Research* (2005) found that individuals who spent more time in deep sleep had healthier body compositions and were likelier to lose fat over time. Conversely, poor sleep leads to muscle breakdown and fat retention, making weight loss more difficult.

Your body continues to burn calories during sleep to maintain essential functions like breathing, circulation, and cellular repair, known as your basal metabolic rate (BMR). During deep sleep (slow-wave sleep), the body releases growth hormone, which aids in fat metabolism and muscle repair. Increased muscle mass, in turn, raises your metabolic rate, allowing you to burn more calories even while at rest.

One often overlooked factor in nighttime fat burning is room temperature. Research has shown that sleeping in a cooler environment can stimulate the body to burn more calories by activating brown adipose tissue (BAT), also known as brown fat.

Unlike white fat, which stores energy, brown fat burns calories to generate heat and maintain body temperature.

A pivotal study by the National Institutes of Health (2014) found that participants who slept in a 66°F (19°C) room for four weeks doubled their brown fat volume and significantly increased their metabolic rate. This increase in brown fat activity led to greater calorie burning during sleep and improved insulin sensitivity, which is crucial for weight management. Conversely, sleeping in warmer environments reduced brown fat activation, limiting these metabolic benefits.

Sleep also regulates cortisol, the body's primary stress hormone. Elevated cortisol levels, especially in the evening, promote fat storage—particularly visceral fat around the abdomen. A study from the University of California, Berkeley (2013) found that poor sleep increases cortisol production, increasing fat accumulation and cravings for high-calorie foods. By prioritizing restful sleep, you can help keep cortisol levels in check, making it easier for your body to burn fat rather than store it.

STRATEGIES TO MAXIMIZE FAT BURNING WHILE YOU SLEEP

To take full advantage of sleep's fat-burning potential, focus on improving both the quality of your sleep and your sleep environment. Aim for 7–9 hours of sleep per night, as the National Sleep Foundation recommends.

1. **Optimize Your Room Temperature:** Keep your bedroom cool, ideally between 60–67°F (15–19°C). Cooler temperatures stimulate brown fat activity, increasing calorie burn throughout the night.

2. **Stick to a Consistent Sleep Schedule:** Going to bed and waking up at the same time every day helps regulate your circadian rhythm, optimizing hormone production and metabolism.

3. **Avoid Late-Night Eating:** Eating heavy meals close to bedtime can disrupt your metabolism and sleep quality. Research in *Cell Metabolism* (2012) suggests that time-restricted eating, in which food intake is limited to a specific window during the day, improves sleep and supports fat loss.

4. **Incorporate Strength Training:** Building muscle increases your resting metabolic rate, allowing you to burn more calories even during sleep. A study in *The Journal of Strength and Conditioning Research* (2015) found that resistance training improved sleep quality and enhanced fat oxidation overnight.

5. **Manage Stress Before Bed:** Practice relaxation techniques like deep breathing or meditation to reduce cortisol levels and promote restful, fat-burning sleep.

UNDERSTANDING SLEEP AND MENTAL HEALTH

Sleep and mental health are deeply interconnected, influencing each other in ways that can enhance or hinder our well-being. Sleeping poorly often feels like a fog descends on your mind, clouding your thoughts and emotions. This isn't just an inconvenience; it's a sign of sleep's profound impact on your mental health. Sleep deprivation is closely linked to mood disorders such as depression. Lack of rest can exacerbate feelings of sadness or hopelessness, pushing you toward a downward spiral that's hard to escape. Conversely, when your mind is overwhelmed with anxiety, falling asleep can become a nightly battle. The worries that linger in your thoughts make it difficult to relax, delaying sleep onset and diminishing its quality.

Mental health challenges frequently manifest themselves in sleep disturbances. Nighttime panic attacks are another burden for many, leaving you suddenly awake with a racing heart and a sense of dread. These episodes can shatter the tranquility of the night, leaving you anxious about sleep itself, which only fuels the problem. Recognizing these patterns is the first step toward addressing them and reclaiming restful nights.

Improving your mental health through better sleep involves practical strategies addressing the mind and body. As described earlier, Cognitive behavioral therapy for insomnia (CBT-I) and mindfulness are highly effective approaches.

Sometimes, the challenges of sleep and mental health require more than self-help strategies. It's important to recognize when professional help is needed. A mental health specialist can provide the support and guidance needed to navigate these issues. Therapy and counseling offer a safe space to explore the underlying causes of your sleep troubles and develop coping mechanisms tailored to your individual needs.

SEASONAL SLEEP ADJUSTMENTS

As the year unfolds, the changing seasons bring about shifts in daylight and weather, which can significantly affect your sleep patterns. These natural transitions can either enhance or hinder your ability to get a good night's sleep, depending on how well you manage them. In winter, longer nights and shorter days can affect your mood and energy levels, often leading to a condition known as seasonal affective disorder or winter blues. The reduced exposure to sunlight disrupts your body's production of serotonin, the hormone that contributes to feelings of well-being and happiness, while also affecting melatonin levels, which regulate sleep. This hormonal imbalance can lead to increased sleepiness during the day and difficulty sleeping at night.

It's crucial to adapt your sleep habits proactively to combat these seasonal changes. Light therapy is powerful for managing winter blues and maintaining a regular sleep schedule. Using a light therapy box that mimics natural daylight can increase your exposure to light during the darker months, helping to regulate your body's internal clock. Placing the lightbox in your morning routine can help signal to your brain that it's time to wake up and be alert, counteracting the effects of shorter days. Additionally, making a conscious effort to spend time outdoors during daylight hours, whether walking during lunch or simply sitting by a window, can help boost your mood and energy levels.

Proactive planning for seasonal transitions can minimize disruptions and help you maintain a stable sleep pattern year-round. For example, adjusting your bedtime routine with daylight savings can ease the transition and reduce the impact on your sleep. You might consider gradually altering your sleep schedule by 10–15 minutes each night in the weeks leading up to the shift. This gradual approach allows your body to acclimate more smoothly, reducing the likelihood of sleep disturbances. By anticipating and accommodating these seasonal changes, you can protect your sleep quality and enjoy restful nights, regardless of the time of year.

Summary:

- **Use Sleep Tracking Tools** – Leverage wearables like smartwatches or apps (e.g., Oura Ring, Google Watch) to monitor sleep cycles, heart rate, and nighttime awakenings. Analyze patterns regularly to identify and address sleep disruptions.

- **Maintain a Sleep Journal** – Complement digital tracking with a handwritten journal to record lifestyle factors influencing sleep. Set monthly goals based on your insights to refine your sleep habits continuously.

- **Explore Virtual Sleep Coaches** – Utilize apps like Sleepio, BetterSleep, or Somryst to access CBT-I-based techniques and personalized feedback for improving sleep. These platforms offer guided exercises and behavior modification strategies.

- **Integrate Sleep with Wellness** – Coordinate exercise, nutrition, and mental health practices to create a positive feedback loop. Regular physical activity, stress management techniques, and mindful eating all contribute to better sleep quality.

- **Maximize Fat Burning During Sleep** – To activate brown fat, optimize your sleep environment by lowering the room temperature (60–67°F). Maintain consistent sleep schedules, manage stress, and avoid late-night eating to support metabolism.

- **Recognize Sleep's Impact on Mental Health** – Address anxiety, depression, and nighttime panic attacks by incorporating CBT-I, mindfulness practices, and, when necessary, professional mental health support to break the cycle of poor sleep and emotional distress.

- **Adjust for Seasonal Changes** – Use light therapy and gradual sleep schedule shifts to combat the effects of shorter days or daylight savings. Spending time outdoors and adjusting routines can minimize seasonal sleep disruptions.

CONCLUSION

"Optimizing sleep isn't about quick fixes—it's about creating sustainable habits that support lifelong health."

— ARIANNA HUFFINGTON (*FOUNDER OF THE SLEEP REVOLUTION*)

As we end this journey, I want to express gratitude for joining me in exploring the transformative power of sleep. Together, we've delved into the science behind slumber, uncovering the core principles that can revolutionize how you approach rest. By understanding the intricacies of sleep stages, circadian rhythms, and the profound impact of sleep on our overall well-being, you've armed yourself with the knowledge to take control of your nights and, consequently, your days.

Throughout these pages, I've emphasized the significance of creating a sleep-friendly environment. This sanctuary invites relaxation and promotes deep, restorative rest. From optimizing your bedroom's temperature and lighting to incorporating soothing scents and sounds, you now possess the tools to craft a space that works harmoniously with your body's natural sleep needs. Remember, small changes can yield remarkable results, and by prioritizing a sleep-conducive environment, you set the stage for a more restful and rejuvenating experience.

Beyond the physical space, we've explored the critical role of effective sleep habits in enhancing sleep quality. Consistency is key, and by establishing a regular sleep routine, you signal to your body that it's time to wind down and prepare for slumber. Equally important are your choices throughout the day—from the foods you eat to how you move your body. By nourishing yourself with sleep-supportive nutrients and engaging in regular physical activity, you create a solid foundation for better sleep and improved overall health.

As you reflect on the insights gained, you will want to focus on the key takeaways that resonated with you most. Review the summaries of each chapter to engrain further some of the simple actions you can take to take charge of your health.

Whether it's the power of mindfulness in quieting a racing mind, the impact of technology on sleep, or the strategies for overcoming specific challenges like sleep latency or nighttime awakenings, trust that you know how to make meaningful changes. And remember, when it comes to family sleep routines, patience, consistency, and open communication are your greatest allies in fostering healthy sleep habits for everyone under your roof.

Embarking on this sleep optimization journey is not a one-time event but a lifelong commitment to prioritizing rest. Embrace the mindset of continuous learning and adaptation, recognizing that what works for you today may evolve as your life and circumstances change. Be open to experimenting with new strategies, adjusting your approach when needed, and celebrating your progress. Every small victory, every well-rested morning, is a testament to your dedication to your well-being.

As you close this book and step into a world of possibilities, I invite you to take ownership of your sleep health. You have the power to transform your nights and, in turn, elevate every aspect of your life. Start small by implementing one new habit or creating a more inviting sleep environment. Track your progress, noting your energy, mood, and productivity improvements. Most importantly, be kind to yourself and understand that setbacks are a natural part of growth.

Remember, you are not alone on this path. As I have shared my struggles and triumphs with sleep, countless others are on a similar journey. My research found better sleep improvement methods than counting backward from ten thousand.

Seek support when needed, whether from loved ones, healthcare professionals, or the ever-growing community of sleep enthusiasts. We can inspire and uplift one another, sharing our experiences and lessons learned.

As you embark on this transformative journey, I leave you with a final thought: Sleep is not a luxury but a necessity. It is the foundation on which we build our lives, the fuel that propels us toward our dreams. By prioritizing sleep, you invest in your present and future, unlock your full potential, and embrace a life of vitality, clarity, and joy.

So, my friend, here's to your sleep revolution. May your nights be filled with peace, your dreams be sweet, and your days brimming with the energy and enthusiasm only a well-rested mind and body can provide. The journey to better sleep starts now, and I am honored to have been a part of your awakening.

With gratitude and hope, Nathan Caldwell

MAKE A DIFFERENCE

Thank you for joining me on this incredible journey through the world of sleep, or, more importantly, getting a great sleep daily. I hope that you found my book as enlightening and inspiring as I intended it to be. I have a small favor to ask—**a moment of your time for a big impact!**

Could you please leave a review? Sharing your thoughts on Amazon helps guide others who are curious about the exciting possibilities of Biohacking Sleep.

Your review will empower others to navigate the ups and downs of rejuvenating their sleeping habits and enhancing their days with renewed energy. Your review makes it easier for them to discover this book and embark on their own journey of maximizing sleep health.

Leaving a review is quick, but the impact is lasting. Whether it's a detailed account of how you applied the insights from the book or a quick note on what chapter you loved the most, your thoughts are incredibly valuable and greatly appreciated.

Here's a direct link to the review page:

https://amzn.to/3EYQ4nv

Thank you once again for your time and support. Here's to your future of refreshing sleep and healthier days to come—may they be as limitless as your potential to achieve and transform yourself. Keep building and improving your sleep processes to make your own meaningful quality-of-life changes. Most importantly, keep sharing your journey!

Nathen Cadwell

REFERENCES

Hopkins Medicine. (n.d.). *The science of sleep: Understanding what happens when you sleep.* Johns Hopkins Medicine. Retrieved from https://www.hopkinsmedicine. org/health/wellness-and-prevention/the-science-of-sleep-understanding-what-happens-when-you-sleep

Arendt, J. (2003). *Melatonin, circadian rhythms, and sleep. Sleep Medicine Reviews, 7*(1), 25-29. Retrieved from https://pubmed.ncbi.nlm.nih.gov/12670411

Reach Wellness. (n.d.). *Common sleep disruptors and how to sleep better.* Retrieved from https://reachwellness.ca/good-sleep

Altena, E., Micoulaud-Franchi, J. A., Geoffroy, P. A., Sanz-Arigita, E. J., Bioulac, S., & Philip, P. (2023). *The consequences of sleep deprivation on cognitive performance and emotional regulation. Frontiers in Neuroscience, 17,* 10155483. Retrieved from https://pmc.ncbi.nlm.nih.gov/articles/PMC10155483

Fox4KC. (n.d.). *Bedroom color affects sleep time and quality, research shows.* Retrieved from https://fox4kc.com/health/bedroom-color-effects-sleep-time-and-quality-research-shows

Sleep Foundation. (n.d.). *The best temperature for sleep.* Retrieved from https://www.sleepfoundation.org/bedroom-environment/best-temperature-for-sleep

Gooley, J. J., Chamberlain, K., Smith, K. A., Khalsa, S. B. S., Rajaratnam, S. M., Van Reen, E., ... Czeisler, C. A. (2011). *Exposure to room light before bedtime suppresses melatonin onset and shortens melatonin duration in humans. Journal of Clinical Endocrinology & Metabolism, 96*(3), E463–E472. Retrieved from https://pmc.ncbi. nlm.nih.gov/articles/PMC3047226

Soundproof Cow. (n.d.). *How to soundproof a bedroom.* Retrieved from https://www. soundproofcow.com/tips-soundproofing-bedroom

ResMed. (n.d.). *7 essential minerals and vitamins for sleep.* Retrieved from https:// www.resmed.co.in/blogs/essential-vitamins-minerals-for-peaceful-sleep

Dashti, H. S., Daghlas, I., Lane, J. M., et al. (2021). *Meal timing, sleep, and cardiometabolic outcomes. Current Opinion in Endocrinology, Diabetes, and Obesity, 28*(1), 45-52. Retrieved from https://www.sciencedirect.com/science/article/abs/pii/S2451965021000247

Mayo Clinic. (n.d.). *Valerian: A safe and effective herbal sleep aid?* Retrieved from https://www.mayoclinic.org/diseases-conditions/insomnia/expert-answers/valerian/faq-20057875

Grandner, M. A., Jackson, N., Gerstner, J. R., & Knutson, K. L. (2014). *Dietary behav-*

iors and poor sleep quality among young adults. Journal of Sleep Research, 23(1), 48-55. Retrieved from https://pmc.ncbi.nlm.nih.gov/articles/PMC7176518

Sleep Health Foundation. (n.d.). *Mindfulness and sleep.* Retrieved from https://www.sleephealthfoundation.org.au/sleep-topics/mindfulness-and-sleep

Medical News Today. (n.d.). *4-7-8 breathing: How it works, benefits, and uses.* Retrieved from https://www.medicalnewstoday.com/articles/324417

WebMD. (n.d.). *Progressive muscle relaxation for stress and insomnia.* Retrieved from https://www.webmd.com/sleep-disorders/muscle-relaxation-for-stress-insomnia

Verywell Mind. (n.d.). *How to use visualization to reduce anxiety symptoms.* Retrieved from https://www.verywellmind.com/visualization-for-relaxation-2584112

Mindell, J. A., et al. (2019). *Implementation of a nightly bedtime routine: How quickly does bedtime behavior improve sleep in young children? Journal of Clinical Sleep Medicine, 15*(5), 749-757. Retrieved from https://pmc.ncbi.nlm.nih.gov/articles/PMC6587179

Clear, J. (n.d.). *How long does it take to form a habit? Backed by science.* Retrieved from https://jamesclear.com/new-habit

National Sleep Foundation. (n.d.). *Sleep debt: The hidden cost of insufficient rest.* Retrieved from https://www.sleepfoundation.org/how-sleep-works/sleep-debt-and-catch-up-sleep

National Heart, Lung, and Blood Institute. (n.d.). *Sleep apnea – Treatment.* Retrieved from https://www.nhlbi.nih.gov/health/sleep-apnea/treatment

NPR. (2021). *How to create a healthy sleep routine: Life Kit.* Retrieved from https://www.npr.org/2021/11/04/1052302645/sleep-routine-children-healthy-building

Hopkins Medicine. (n.d.). *New parents: Tips for quality rest.* Retrieved from https://www.hopkinsmedicine.org/health/wellness-and-prevention/new-parents-tips-for-quality-rest

www.ingramcontent.com/pod-product-compliance
Lightning Source LLC
Chambersburg PA
CBHW070119030426
42335CB00016B/2204